MOSBY'S

Fluids & Electrolytes
Memory
NoteCards

Visual, Mnemonic, and
Memory Aids for Nurses

JoAnn Zerwekh, EdD, RN, FNP, APRN, BC
Executive Director　　**Nursing Faculty – Online Campus**
Nursing Education Consultants　　University of Phoenix
Ingram, Texas　　Phoenix, Arizona

Jo Carol Claborn, MS, RN, CNS
Executive Director
Nursing Education Consultants
Ingram, Texas

Tom Gaglione, RN, MSN
Nursing Faculty
Nursing Education Consultants
Ingram, Texas

CJ Miller, BSN, RN

**With the collaboration
of Ashley Zerwekh, RN, BA**

MOSBY
ELSEVIER

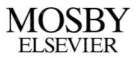

MOSBY
ELSEVIER

11830 Westline Industrial Drive
St. Louis, Missouri 63146

MOSBY'S FLUIDS & ELECTROLYTES   ISBN-10: 0-323-03725-9
MEMORY NOTECARDS: VISUAL,   ISBN-13: 978-0-323-03725-9
MNEMONIC, AND MEMORY AIDS
FOR NURSES
Copyright © 2006, Mosby, Inc. All rights reserved.

NOTICE

Nursing is an ever-changing field. Standard safety precautions must be followed, but as new research and clinical experience broaden our knowledge, changes in treatment and drug therapy may become necessary or appropriate. Readers are advised to check the most current product information provided by the manufacturer of each drug to be administered to verify the recommended dose, the method and duration of administration, and contraindications. It is the responsibility of the licensed prescriber, relying on experience and knowledge of the patient, to determine dosages and the best treatment for each individual patient. Neither the publisher nor the editor assumes any liability for any injury and/or damage to persons or property arising from this publication.

ISBN-10: 0-323-03725-9
ISBN-13: 978-0-323-03725-9

Executive Publisher: Robin Carter
Developmental Editor: Jamie Horn
Book Production Manager: Gayle May
Senior Book Designer: Julia Dummitt
Cover Art: CJ Miller

Printed in China.

Contents

FLUIDS & ELECTROLYTES

ACID-BASE BALANCE

IMPORTANT BODY MINERALS

IV THERAPY

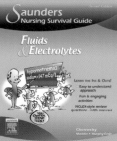

FINALLY, FLUIDS AND ELECTROLYTES MADE CLEAR! USE YOUR NEW MEMORY NOTECARDS AS A:

- Pocket reference for clinicals
- Companion study guide for medical-surgical and fluids and electrolytes texts
- Quick review for exams
- Patient teaching aid
- Resource for writing nursing care plans

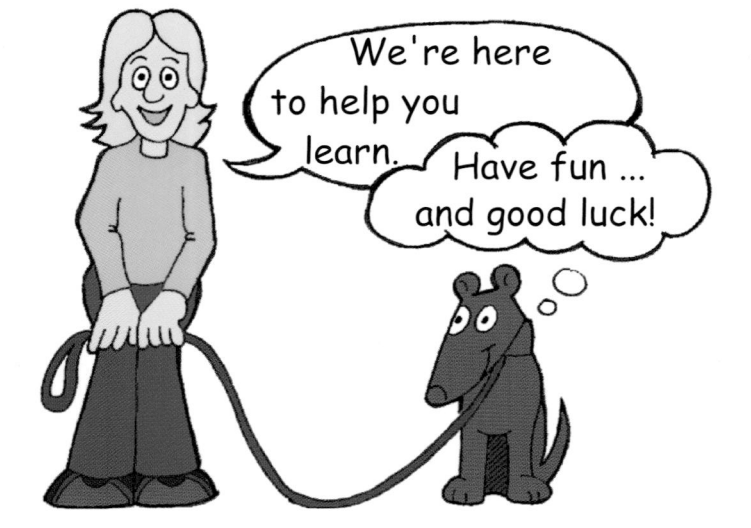

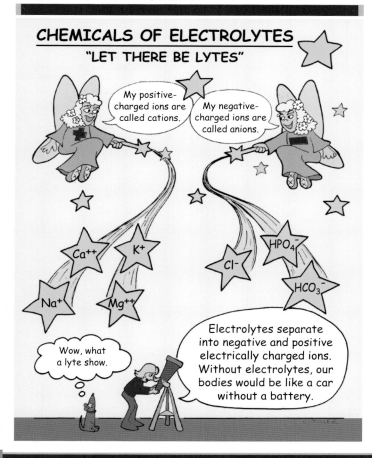

Electrolyte Overview

SIGNIFICANCE OF ELECTROLYTES

Electrolytes are substances found in the intracellular (ICF) and extracellular fluid (ECF) whose molecules split into ions when placed in water. The major electrolytes found in the body are potassium, sodium, calcium, chloride, phosphorous, and magnesium. Electrolytes are distinguished by their electrical charge as either positive or negative. Electrolytes that have a positive charge are known as *cations*. Electrolytes that have a negative charge are known as *anions*. Examples of cations are potassium, sodium, magnesium, and calcium. Examples of anions are bicarbonate, chloride, and phosphate. Without electrolytes, the body cannot maintain homeostasis.

SOURCES OF ELECTROLYTES

Can be found in certain foods:

- Fruits, vegetables, and grains
- Red meat, poultry, and fish
- Fluids
- Supplements

CONTROL OF ELECTROLYTES

Electrolytes are regulated in the body by their degree of concentration. Diffusion, active transport, and osmosis are mechanisms that maintain electrolyte balance in the body.

Diffusion is a process that moves molecules from an area of higher concentration to an area of lower concentration. No energy is required.

Active transport occurs when molecules move across the concentration gradient. An example of this is the sodium-potassium pump. Sodium moves out of the cell as potassium moves into the cell to maintain a steady concentration balance. Adenosine triphosphate is the energy required for this process.

Osmosis is the process in which water moves from a dilute area (area containing more water) to an area that has less water.

FUNCTIONS OF ELECTROLYTES

- Maintain homeostasis
- Fluid regulation
- Acid-base regulation

Common clinical findings	Patient teaching
Important nursing implications	Serious/life-threatening implications

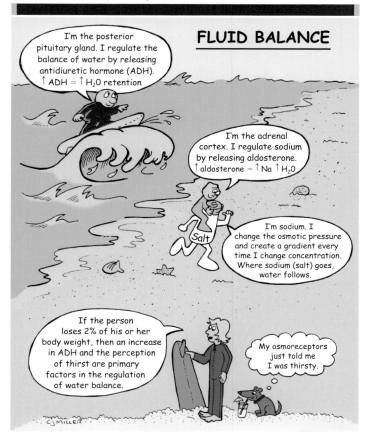

— What You Need to Know —
Overview of Fluid Balance

SIGNIFICANCE OF FLUID BALANCE

Water makes up about 60% of our body weight. It is the necessary component in maintaining homeostasis.

SOURCES OF FLUIDS

- Water and any other liquid that can be ingested
- IV fluids (0.9% normal saline [NS], 5% dextrose in 0.45% NS, or albumin)
- Fruits, vegetables, lean meats

CONTROL OF FLUIDS

Fluid balance is regulated in the body by the body's own thirst mechanism, the hypothalamus, the pituitary and adrenal glands, the kidneys, and the gastrointestinal (GI) system. Insensible water loss or fluid that cannot be measured accounts for about 900 ml of fluid loss in an adult per day.

Thirst mechanism is initiated when a person's body fluid decreases. Osmoreceptors in the hypothalamus initiate a stimulus that senses a need for fluids.

The hypothalamus makes ADH, and the posterior pituitary gland stores the ADH until the hypothalamus initiates a signal to the pituitary gland, causing ADH to be released. Once ADH is released in the body, the distal tubules of the kidneys respond by reabsorbing water. Therefore after a person drinks a glass of water, ADH prevents it from becoming excreted.

The adrenal cortex secretes aldosterone (mineralocorticoid), which has properties of sodium reabsorption and potassium excretion. Remember, water follows salt. As sodium is reabsorbed, water follows as a result of osmotic change.

The kidneys regulate fluid balance by adjusting the amount of urine volume that is excreted. An adult excretes 1.5 L of urine per day on average.

The GI tract is responsible for absorbing water intake. A small amount of fluid is lost in feces. However, diarrhea and vomiting can cause major fluid volume deficits.

Common clinical findings	Patient teaching
Important nursing implications	Serious/life-threatening implications

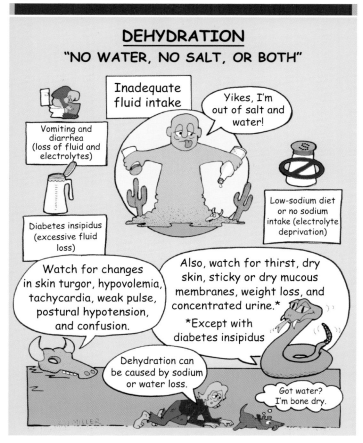

What You Need to Know
Dehydration (Fluid Deficit)

GENERAL

Dehydration occurs when fluid intake is less than fluid output. Dehydration can be caused by inadequate intake of fluids or hyperexcretion of fluids as in the case of diarrhea or vomiting.

SIGNS AND SYMPTOMS

Moderate
- Flushed dry skin
- Dry mucous membranes, tenting (skin turgor), decreased urine output
- Urine characteristics: ↑specific gravity, color may be dark yellow to amber
- Thirst and weight loss
- Client may be restless, lethargic

Severe Deficit
- Skin may be cold and clammy
- Dry, cracked tongue
- Soft, sunken eyeballs
- Thready pulse, tachycardia
- Postural hypotension, rapid respiratory rate
- Lethargy progressing to coma
- Absence of tearing or sweating
- Oliguric or very concentrated urine
- Hemoconcentration—↑Hct, blood urea nitrogen (BUN), electrolytes

DIAGNOSTIC FINDINGS
- Urine specific gravity >1.020
- Elevated H&H
- Elevated potassium levels

Common clinical findings   Patient teaching

Important nursing implications   Serious/life-threatening implications

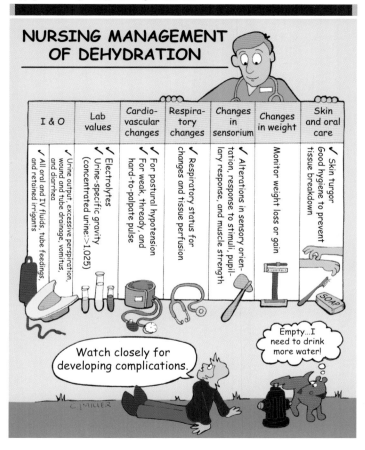

What You Need to Know
Management of Dehydration

MEDICAL MANAGEMENT

- The goal of treatment is to restore fluid loss.
- IV fluids will be determined depending on the severity of sodium loss associated with dehydration.
- Isotonic solutions are usually used in the initial treatment.

NURSING MANAGEMENT

- Identify clients at increased risk for fluid volume deficit.
- Monitor vital signs. (Assess for postural hypotension.)
- Measure total intake and output (I&O) and document it.
- Obtain accurate daily weights.
- Skin turgor is a poor indication of hydration status in the elderly.
- Evaluate urinary output and specific gravity.
- Monitor serum laboratory values for concentrations of Hct, BUN, and sodium.
- Monitor hemoglobin and hematocrit (H&H) levels.
- Hypovolemic shock is a serious complication associated with dehydration as a result of inadequate blood volume to maintain normal circulation.
- Assess client's level of consciousness.
- Change in mentation may occur in severe dehydration.
- Evaluate the client's response to fluid replacement.
- Encourage the client to increase oral intake before doing any strenuous activity.
- Teach the client the importance of consuming at least 64 oz of water daily to prevent dehydration.

| Common clinical findings | Patient teaching |
| Important nursing implications | Serious/life-threatening implications |

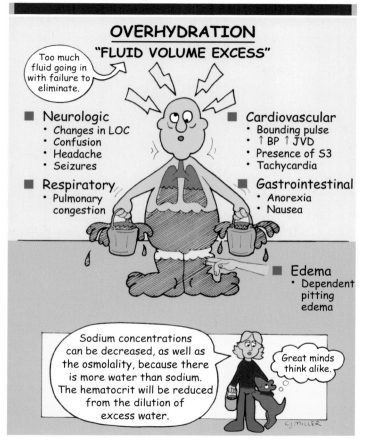

What You Need to Know
Overhydration (Fluid Volume Excess)

GENERAL

When the body (kidneys, liver, heart) is functioning normally, it is difficult for the body to have an excess of fluids. When excess water is retained, it causes a dilution of the ECF and water moves into the ICF. Overhydration is caused by excessive fluid in the ECF.

Overhydration is also called *hypotonic hydration* or *water intoxication*.

Overhydration may also be caused by rapid infusion of IV fluids.

Edema may exist in states of overhydration, but edema and overhydration are not the same. Do not assume that edema indicates overhydration.

SIGNS AND SYMPTOMS

- Edema—peripheral pitting
- Positive jugular vein distention (JVD)
- Respiratory difficulty, shortness of breath (SOB), moist breath sounds, coughing
- Weight gain
- Mental confusion, lethargy
- Muscular cramping
- Nausea
- Cerebral edema

DIAGNOSTIC FINDINGS

- Hyponatremia (serum sodium level <135 mEq/L)
- Decreased specific gravity
- Low H&H levels

Common clinical findings	Patient teaching
Important nursing implications	Serious/life-threatening implications

NURSING MANAGEMENT OF OVERHYDRATION

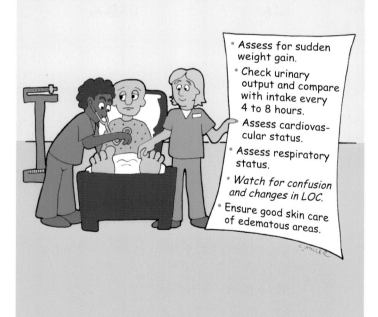

- Assess for sudden weight gain.
- Check urinary output and compare with intake every 4 to 8 hours.
- Assess cardiovascular status.
- Assess respiratory status.
- Watch for confusion and changes in LOC.
- Ensure good skin care of edematous areas.

What You Need to Know
Management of Overhydration

MEDICAL MANAGEMENT
- The goal is to decrease the amount of fluid in the cells.
- Hypertonic solution may be given.
- Mannitol is the diuretic of choice because of its osmotic properties. Its action works by reversing the osmotic gradient and pulling water out of the cell.

NURSING MANAGEMENT
- Monitor the client for a change in mentation.
  - Change in mentation is an early sign of cerebral edema.
- Monitor daily weight.
- Monitor I&O.
- Decrease intake of H_2O and Na.
- Elevate the head of the bed.
- Encourage mobility.
- Monitor electrolytes—especially K and Na.
- Assess for history of conditions that may cause fluid retention: heart failure, renal failure, pancreatitis, or high salt intake.
- Teach the client to limit intake of oral fluids.
- Teach the client early signs and symptoms associated with water retention.

Common clinical findings   Patient teaching

Important nursing implications   Serious/life-threatening implications

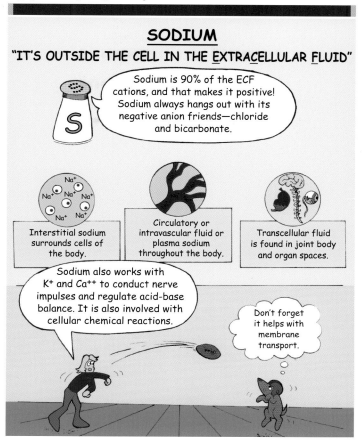

SIGNIFICANCE OF SODIUM

Sodium is the major cation found in the extracellular fluid (ECF), and its role is to maintain fluid volume in the body. The normal laboratory value of sodium is 135 to 145 mEq/L.

SOURCES OF SODIUM

- Table salt, seasonings, spices
- Processed foods
- Hot dogs, cold cuts, beef jerky, canned soup
- Saltine crackers, pretzels, potato chips
- Canned soda beverages
- Pickles and other pickled foods
- Sardines and herring
- Potatoes and other white vegetables

CONTROL OF SODIUM

Sodium is controlled by several mechanisms in the body:

- Osmoreceptors send a message to the brain when too much sodium is in the ECF, and they initiate the thirst mechanism. This causes the person to drink a glass of water to quench his or her thirst.
- The hypothalamus stimulates the pituitary gland to release antidiuretic hormone (ADH). ADH helps to retain body fluids.
- The kidneys will now hold onto this extra fluid in the body to decrease the serum osmolality of the sodium (sodium will follow the water).

FUNCTIONS OF SODIUM

- Regulates osmolality
- Helps maintain blood pressure by balancing the volume of water in the body
- Works with other electrolytes to promote the transmission of nerve impulses to muscles and tissues
- Helps maintain acid-base balance

Common clinical findings   Patient teaching

Important nursing implications   Serious/life-threatening implications

HYPERNATREMIA

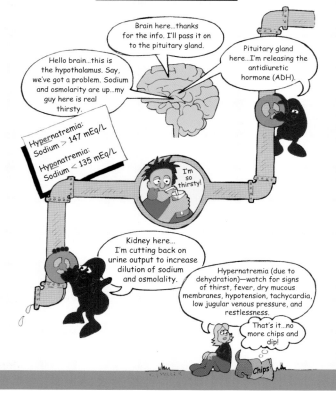

What You Need to Know
Hypernatremia

GENERAL

When serum sodium levels are >145 mEq/L, hypernatremia is the condition that results. Hypernatremia may result from several problems:

- Dehydration—causes an increase in the concentration of the sodium in the serum
- Excessive sodium intake
- Interruption of the body's regulatory mechanism for sodium

Hypernatremia can occur from many factors such as eating a high-sodium meal, not drinking enough fluids, leading to dehydration, or administering IV fluids that are considered hypertonic (0.9% NS, $D_5$1/2 in NS, or sodium bicarbonate).

Some other disease processes that can interrupt the body's sodium regulatory mechanism are diabetes insipidus, renal failure, hyperaldosteronism, Cushing's syndrome, and hyperosmolar hyperglycemia nonketotic (HHNK).

Medications that promote osmotic diuresis (mannitol) may also cause hypernatremia—fluid is lost and the sodium is concentrated.

SIGNS AND SYMPTOMS

- Irritability, restlessness, confusion, twitching
- Increased thirst, dry mucous membranes
- Decreased urinary output
- Dyspnea or pulmonary edema from sodium gain
- Flushed skin
- Orthostatic hypotension (fluid loss)

DIAGNOSTIC FINDINGS

- Serum sodium >145 mEq/L
- Serum osmolality >300 mOsm/kg
- Specific gravity >1.030

HEMODYNAMIC MEASUREMENTS

- Sodium excess—↑ CVP and PAP
- Water loss—↓ CVP and PAP

Common clinical findings	Patient teaching
Important nursing implications	Serious/life-threatening implications

HYPERNATREMIA
"YOU ARE FRIED"

F Fever (low grade), flushed skin

R Restless (irritable)

I Increased fluid retention and ↑ BP

E Edema (peripheral and pitting)

D Decreased urine output, dry mouth

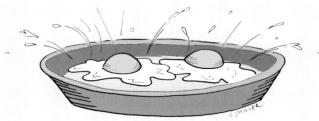

Hypernatremia—FRIED

The acronym FRIED is a mnemonic to help you remember the signs and symptoms of hypernatremia. Think of the body heat of the fever and the heat of a frying pan—the visual image will help you associate the two.

GENERAL

When serum sodium levels are >145 mEq/L, hypernatremia is the condition that results. It most often occurs when there is a decrease in water intake leading to an increased sodium concentration.

SIGNS AND SYMPTOMS

- **F**ever (low grade), flushed skin
- **R**estlessness, irritability, confusion
- **I**ncreased fluid retention, increased BP
- **E**dema (peripheral and pitting)
- **D**ecreased urinary output, dry mouth, increased thirst
- Twitching
- Dyspnea

Common clinical findings	Patient teaching
Important nursing implications	Serious/life-threatening implications

HYPERNATREMIA
"THE MODEL"
(Causes of ↑ serum sodium)

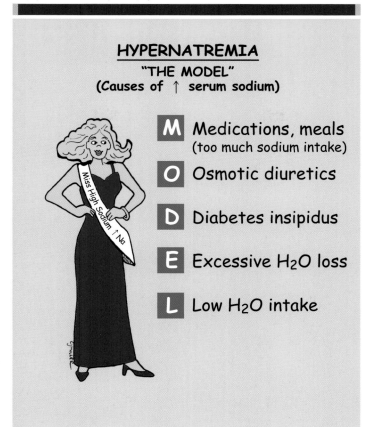

M Medications, meals
(too much sodium intake)

O Osmotic diuretics

D Diabetes insipidus

E Excessive H$_2$O loss

L Low H$_2$O intake

GENERAL

The acronym MODEL emphasizes **M**edication and meals, **O**smotic diuretics, **D**iabetes insipidus, **E**xcessive water loss, and **L**ow water intake. The trick is to mentally attach the picture and the acronym to the symptoms to enhance memory recall.

When serum sodium levels are >145 mEq/L, hypernatremia is the condition that results.

Hypernatremia can be caused by many factors such as eating a high-sodium meal, not drinking enough fluids leading to dehydration, or administering IV fluids that are considered hypertonic (0.9% NS, $D_5$1/2 in NS, or sodium bicarbonate).

Some other disease processes that can cause hypernatremia are diabetes insipidus, renal failure, hyperaldosteronism, Cushing's syndrome, and HHNK.

Medications that promote osmotic diuresis (mannitol) may also cause hypernatremia.

CAUSES OF HYPERNATREMIA

- **M**edications and meals (too much salt intake)
- **O**smotic diuretics
- **D**iabetes insipidus
- **E**xcessive water loss
- **L**ow water intake

Common clinical findings   Patient teaching

Important nursing implications   Serious/life-threatening implications

---

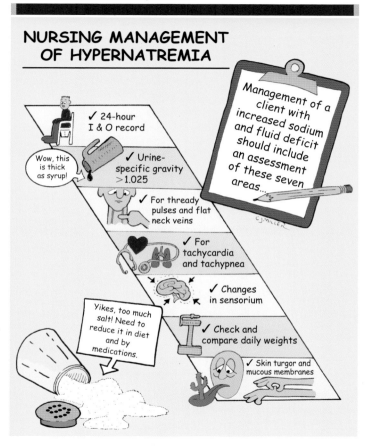

═══ What You Need to Know ═══
Management of Hypernatremia

Treatment depends on the cause of the hypernatremia—either water lost or sodium gained. Corrections should be done slowly to avoid shift of water into the cerebral cells.

MEDICAL MANAGEMENT
- Diuretic therapy to promote excretion of sodium
  - Lasix may be given.
- Hydration therapy
  - Sodium-free isotonic fluids, like D_5W (5% dextrose in water) help dilute the serum sodium followed with 0.45% NS to prevent hyponatremia.
- Treat underlying cause
  - If caused by too rapid infusion of hypertonic solution, the physician may decrease the rate.
  - Ask the client about his or her daily diet (high sodium–containing foods may be a contributing cause).
  - If the client is dehydrated, provide fluids.

NURSING MANAGEMENT
- Monitor vital signs.
  - Tachycardia
  - Blood pressure high with fluid overload and decreased with fluid deficit
  - Increased temperature >101° F
- Measure intake and output.
- Obtain daily weight (before breakfast or same time each day).
  - Make sure the client is wearing the same type of clothes from the previous day and use the same scale.
  - Inform the client that a weight gain of 2 lb or greater in a 4-day period should be reported to the physician immediately.
  - A loss of 4.4 lb is approximately a loss of 2 L fluid.
- Assess for edema in the peripheral extremities, sacrum, and in the face.
- Monitor the client for risk of seizures.

Common clinical findings	Patient teaching
Important nursing implications	Serious/life-threatening implications

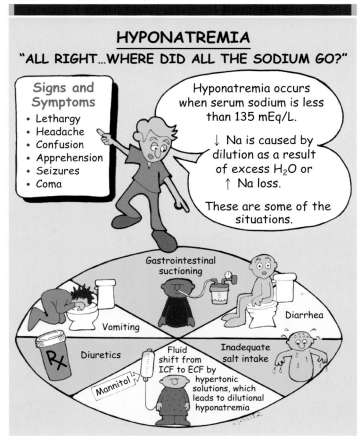

What You Need to Know
Hyponatremia

GENERAL

When serum sodium concentration in the body decreases, the condition is known as *hyponatremia*. Hyponatremia may be caused by excessive dilution of the sodium by overhydration or by an increase in sodium loss from the body. Hyponatremia is serum sodium level <135 mEq/L. With hyponatremia of <125 mEq/L, an intracellular fluid (ICF) shift may occur that will result in cerebral edema and intracranial pressure (ICP).

The following may cause hyponatremia:
- Most common cause is IV fluid overload with inappropriate use of sodium-free or hypotonic IV fluids (fluid gain)
- Fluid overload after drinking water (fluid gain)
- Dilutional states (hyperglycemia and syndrome of inappropriate ADH [SIADH], congestive heart failure [CHF]) (fluid gain)
- Aggressive diuretic therapy (sodium lost)
- GI drainage, diarrhea, vomiting, fistulas (sodium lost)
- Excessive sweating (sodium lost)

SIGNS AND SYMPTOMS

Sodium Loss
- Irritability, apprehension, confusion
- Postural hypotension, tachycardia
- ↓CVP, ↓jugular vein filling
- Weight loss, dry mucous membranes
- Tremors, seizures, coma
- <125 mEq/L (Assess neurologic signs for ICP and cerebral edema.)

Water Gain
- Headache, apathy, confusion
- Weight gain, ↑blood pressure, ↑CVP
- Hallmark sign: nausea, vomiting, anorexia, lethargy, and weakness
- Increased urinary output
- Cerebral edema more common in pediatrics

DIAGNOSTIC FINDINGS
- Serum sodium <135 mEq/L
- Urine specific gravity <1.010
- Critical level <110 mEq/L

Common clinical findings	Patient teaching
Important nursing implications	Serious/life-threatening implications

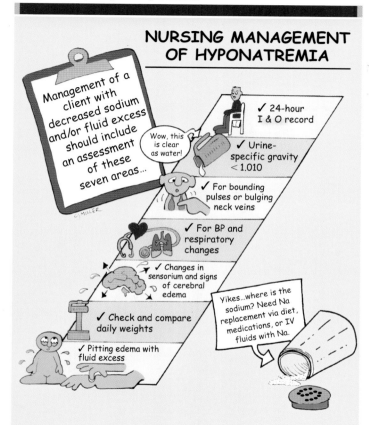

Management of Hyponatremia

MEDICAL MANAGEMENT

- Treat the underlying cause.
- Administer hypertonic saline solutions to restore sodium balance 0.45% NS or D_5 in 0.45% NS.
- Too rapid correction of sodium can cause irreversible neurologic damage.
- Provide nutritional counseling and increase foods containing sodium.

NURSING MANAGEMENT

- Closely monitor neurologic signs during sodium replacement.
- Obtain daily weights.
- Measure I&O—loss or gain of 4.4 lb is equal to 2 L of fluid.
- Check the color, consistency, and amount of urine. The urine should be a light straw color without sediment present.
- Monitor vital signs.
- Assess for intravascular overload during infusion of sodium solutions—tachypnea, tachycardia, SOB.
- Teach the client how much fluid he or she is allowed per day and how to identify fluid retention.

Common clinical findings   Patient teaching

Important nursing implications   Serious/life-threatening implications

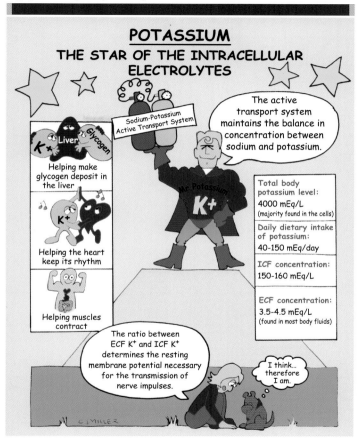

What You Need to Know
Potassium

SIGNIFICANCE OF POTASSIUM

Potassium is the most abundant cation found in intracellular fluid (ICF). Potassium regulates fluid balance and keeps osmolality within the ICF. Potassium also plays a key role in preserving normal cardiac rhythms and maintaining skeletal and smooth muscle contraction. Changes in serum pH also precipitate changes in serum potassium.

SOURCES OF POTASSIUM

- Bananas, dark green leafy vegetables, raisins, salt-substitutes
- All-bran cereal, potatoes, and dried beef (beef jerky, deer meat)

CONTROL OF POTASSIUM

Kidneys are the primary regulators of potassium. As the serum potassium level rises, so does the level in the renal tubules. A concentration gradient occurs and potassium is lost in the urine.

Too much potassium in the extracellular fluid (ECF) increases catecholamine levels, causing aldosterone levels to increase. Increased aldosterone levels cause the potassium to leave the ECF and travel into the kidneys (distal renal tubules), where it is excreted with urine.

Insulin can also lower the concentration of potassium by helping potassium travel into liver and muscle cells where it is used in the process of breaking down carbohydrates and proteins by moving glucose into the ICF.

Clients receiving increased amounts of insulin (TPN, DKA) should have potassium levels monitored closely because insulin may cause low levels of potassium.

FUNCTIONS OF POTASSIUM

- Maintains fluid balance in the cells
- Skeletal, cardiac, and smooth muscle contraction
- Helps breakdown carbohydrates and fats
- Promotes cellular growth
- Maintains acid-base balance

Common clinical findings   Patient teaching

Important nursing implications   Serious/life-threatening implications

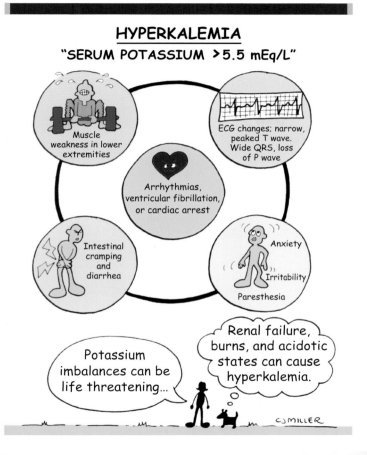

Hyperkalemia

GENERAL

The normal serum potassium level is 3.5 to 5.0 mEq/L. When the potassium level is >5.1 mEq/L, the condition is known as *hyperkalemia*. Hyperkalemia most commonly occurs as a result of excessive potassium intake combined with the body's inability to excrete potassium.

Acute renal failure, Addison's disease, and interstitial nephritis secondary to diabetes mellitus will decrease the excretion of potassium.

Ingestion of potassium-containing foods in clients with renal failure and administration of IV potassium may also cause increased serum potassium levels.

SIGNS AND SYMPTOMS

- Muscle cramps in the lower extremities followed by weakness
- Diarrhea, hyperactive bowel sounds
- Numbness and tingling in the extremities
- Lethargy and fatigue
- Bradycardia
- Hypotension
- Cardiac arrhythmias
- Electrocardiographic (ECG) changes
  - Peaked T wave
  - Wide and bizarre QRS complex
  - Prolonged QT intervals (potassium >8 mEq/L)

DIAGNOSTIC FINDINGS

- Serum potassium >5.1 mEq/L

| Common clinical findings | Patient teaching |
| Important nursing implications | Serious/life-threatening implications |

<u>MURDER</u>

SIGNS AND SYMPTOMS OF INCREASED SERUM K

M—Muscle weakness

U—Urine, oliguria, anuria

R—Respiratory distress

D—Decreased cardiac contractility

E—ECG changes

R—Reflexes, hyperreflexia, or areflexia (flaccid)

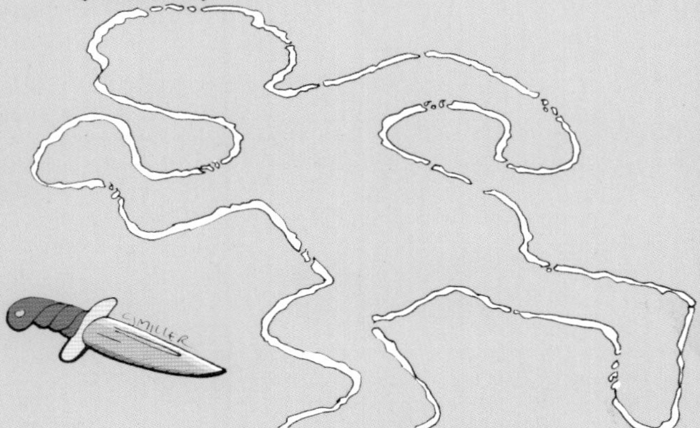

============================== **What You Need to Know** ==============================
Hyperkalemia—MURDER

GENERAL

The normal serum potassium level is 3.5 to 5.0 mEq/L. When the potassium level is >5.1 mEq/L, the condition is known as *hyperkalemia*. Hyperkalemia most commonly occurs as a result of excessive potassium intake combined with the body's inability to excrete potassium.

Use the acronym MURDER to trigger the symptoms that go with each letter of the word—**M**uscle weakness, **U**rine, **R**espiratory distress, **D**ecreased cardiac contractility, **E**CG changes, and **R**eflexes.

SIGNS AND SYMPTOMS

- **M**uscle cramps in the lower extremities followed by weakness
- **U**rine, oliguria, anuria
- **R**espiratory distress
- **D**ecreased cardiac contractility
- **E**CG changes
- **R**eflexes, hyperreflexia or areflexia (flaccid)

| Common clinical findings | Patient teaching |
| Important nursing implications | Serious/life-threatening implications |

THE HYPERKALEMIA "MACHINE"
CAUSES OF INCREASED SERUM K

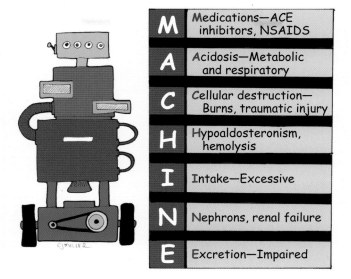

M — Medications—ACE inhibitors, NSAIDS

A — Acidosis—Metabolic and respiratory

C — Cellular destruction—Burns, traumatic injury

H — Hypoaldosteronism, hemolysis

I — Intake—Excessive

N — Nephrons, renal failure

E — Excretion—Impaired

================== **What You Need to Know** ==================
Hyperkalemia—MACHINE

GENERAL

The MACHINE acronym (**M**edication, **A**cidosis, **C**ellular destruction, **H**ypoaldosteronism, **I**ntake, **N**ephrons, **E**xcretion) can be used to trigger memory association with symptoms related to each letter of the word.

The normal serum potassium level is 3.5 to 5.0 mEq/L. When the potassium level is >5.1 mEq/L, the condition is known as *hyperkalemia*. Hyperkalemia most commonly occurs as a result of excessive potassium intake combined with the body's inability to excrete potassium.

CAUSES OF HYERKALEMIA

- **M**edications—angiotensin-converting enzyme (ACE) inhibitors, nonsteroidal antiinflammatory drugs (NSAIDS)
- **A**cidosis—metabolic and respiratory
- **C**ellular destruction—burns, traumatic injury
- **H**ypoaldosteronism, hemolysis
- **I**ntake—excessive
- **N**ephrons—renal failure
- **E**xcretion—impaired

| Common clinical findings | Patient teaching |
| Important nursing implications | Serious/life-threatening implications |

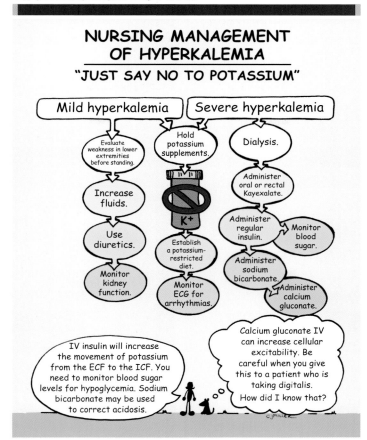

MEDICAL MANAGEMENT

- Eliminate potassium intake, both oral and IV.
- Promote excretion of potassium by administering diuretics.
- Dialysis may be initiated if the client is in renal failure.
- Kayexalate is an ion-exchange resin (it exchanges sodium ions for potassium ions in the intestine and excretes the potassium via the feces) that may be given to treat mild to moderate hyperkalemia.
- IV insulin administration can be given to push potassium from the extracellular fluid (ECF) to the intracellular fluid (ICF). It may be given with glucose to prevent rebound hypoglycemia.
- If hyperkalemia is secondary to acidosis, then IV sodium bicarbonate may be administered.
- IV calcium gluconate may be given immediately to the client experiencing cardiac arrhythmias secondary to life-threatening potassium levels.

NURSING MANAGEMENT

- Assess dietary potassium intake.
- Monitor renal function (urine output, lab values).
- Teach the client that the use of ACE inhibitors and potassium-sparing diuretics will cause increased serum levels of potassium.
- Teach the client to limit the amount of foods containing potassium (leafy vegetables, salt substitutes, dried fruits, bananas, and cantaloupe).
- Teach the client the signs and symptoms of hyperkalemia and about the need to report them to the physician immediately.
- The client will need continuous ECG monitoring while in the hospital to monitor for arrhythmias.
- Monitor BS levels with insulin administration.

Common clinical findings	Patient teaching
Important nursing implications	Serious/life-threatening implications

HYPOKALEMIA

"POTASSIUM IS DANGEROUS WHEN IT IS TOO LOW!"
(SERUM K⁺ < 3.5 mEq/L)

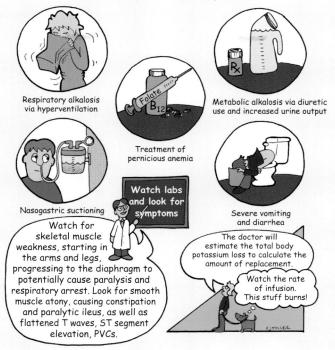

Respiratory alkalosis via hyperventilation

Treatment of pernicious anemia

Metabolic alkalosis via diuretic use and increased urine output

Nasogastric suctioning

Watch labs and look for symptoms

Severe vomiting and diarrhea

Watch for skeletal muscle weakness, starting in the arms and legs, progressing to the diaphragm to potentially cause paralysis and respiratory arrest. Look for smooth muscle atony, causing constipation and paralytic ileus, as well as flattened T waves, ST segment elevation, PVCs.

The doctor will estimate the total body potassium loss to calculate the amount of replacement.

Watch the rate of infusion. This stuff burns!

Hypokalemia

GENERAL

When the serum potassium level is <3.5 mEq/L, the condition is known as *hypokalemia*. The main cause of hypokalemia occurs from abnormal losses in the body, such as diuresis. During diuresis, potassium is excreted with urine as a result of high aldosterone levels. Thiazides and loop diuretics are primary causes of hypokalemia.

A direct relationship exists with low magnesium levels and low potassium levels. Low magnesium levels stimulate the release of renin, which causes an increase in aldosterone levels and excretion of potassium.

GI losses can lower potassium levels, (diarrhea, vomiting, gastric suctioning and ostomy fluids).

Other conditions that may cause low potassium levels are diabetic keto-acidosis, metabolic alkalosis, and pernicious anemia.

SIGNS AND SYMPTOMS

- Fatigue, weakness (early signs)
- Leg cramps
- Weak, irregular pulse
- Polyuria
- Hyperglycemia
- Bradycardia
- ECG changes
  - Flattened T wave
  - ST segment depression
  - Frequent premature ventricular contractions (PVCs)

DIAGNOSTIC FINDINGS

- Serum potassium <3.5 mEq/L

Common clinical findings	Patient teaching
Important nursing implications	Serious/life-threatening implications

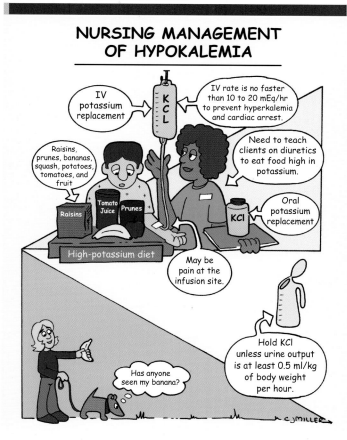

Management of Hypokalemia

MEDICAL MANAGEMENT

- Administration of potassium chloride (KCl) supplements when clients are on loop or thiazide diuretics and digitalis aids in prevention of hypokalemia.
- Potassium may be given orally or IV.
- When given intravenously, potassium may cause irritation and pain at the IV site. Central lines are the preferred site for IV administration.
- The preferred level for serum potassium is 3.5 to 5.0 mEq/L. KCl should be administered IV at a rate of 10 to 20 mEq/L over an hour. Rapid infusion could cause cardiac arrest.
- Hypokalemia will increase the action of digitalis.

NURSING MANAGEMENT

- If given orally, encourage the client to take the KCl supplement with a full glass of water to promote absorption in the GI tract.
- Never give potassium IV push; it may be fatal.
- Monitor the IV site for phlebitis or infiltration; KCl is irritating to the veins.
- Monitor the client on digitalis for signs of digitalis toxicity.
- Teach the client to recognize signs and symptoms of hypokalemia and the need to report them to the physician immediately.
- For clients taking diuretics, explain the importance of increasing potassium intake in the diet.
- Teach the client about foods that are high in potassium.
- Teach the client that salt substitutes contain 50 to 60 mEq/L of potassium and should be avoided if the client is taking a potassium-sparing diuretic.
- Explain the need for a follow-up visit to have serum potassium levels drawn for those at risk.

Common clinical findings	Patient teaching
Important nursing implications	Serious/life-threatening implications

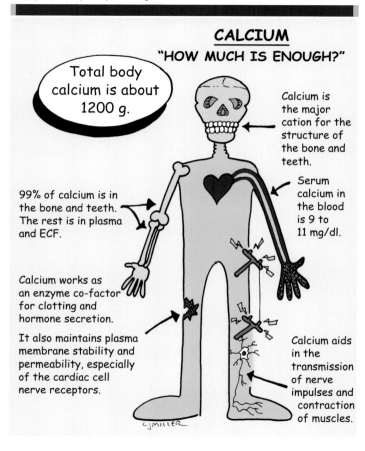

Calcium

SIGNIFICANCE OF CALCIUM

Calcium is commonly found in bones and teeth. It is the most abundant mineral found in the body. Calcium assists with maintenance of muscle tone, hormone secretion, transmission of nerve impulses, and contraction of skeletal and heart muscles.

SOURCES OF CALCIUM

Commonly found in the following products:

- Dairy products—milk, cheese, yogurt, sour cream, cottage cheese, ice cream
- Canned salmon, sardines, oysters
- Fruit juices labeled "fortified"
- Dark green leafy vegetables: spinach, kale, rhubarb, collard greens, broccoli

CONTROL OF CALCIUM

Calcium is controlled by parathyroid hormone (PTH), vitamin D, and calcitonin. PTH is excreted by the parathyroid gland when low levels of serum calcium are present. PTH assists with moving calcium out of the bones, increasing GI reabsorption of calcium in the ileum, and renal tubule reabsorption of calcium. Vitamin D is necessary for absorption of calcium from the GI tract. Calcitonin is produced by the thyroid gland. It is excreted when high levels of serum calcium are found. Calcitonin does the exact opposite of PTH because it is trying to prevent absorption of calcium and promote excretion through the renal tubules. If an increase in calcium exists, then most often a decrease in phosphate is seen, and vice versa.

FUNCTIONS OF CALCIUM

- Necessary for development of strong teeth and bones
- Helps maintain muscle tone
- Contributes to regulation of blood pressure by maintaining cardiac contractility
- Is an enzyme cofactor in the clotting cascade; assists to form blood clots by the release of thromboplastin from platelets
- Necessary for nerve transmission and contraction of skeletal and cardiac muscle

Common clinical findings	Patient teaching
Important nursing implications	Serious/life-threatening implications

HYPERCALCEMIA
"TOO MUCH CALCIUM!"

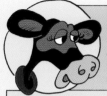

Back with the facts! Serum calcium levels >11mg/dl are too much. It can be the outcome of hyperparathyroidism and bone metastases with calcium resorption from the breast, the lung, or multiple myeloma.

Hypercalcemia causes a loss of excitability in cell membranes and fatigue, weakness, lethargy, anorexia, nausea, constipation, and kidney stones from increased calcium salts.

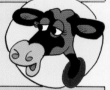

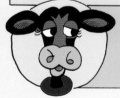

ECG activity may show shortened QT segments and depressed T waves, bradycardia, and varying degrees of heart block.

I want to be a cow when I grow up.

What You Need to Know
Hypercalcemia

GENERAL

Hypercalcemia can be caused by several factors. Increased intake of vitamin D and vitamin A can cause an elevated calcium level. Hyperparathyroidism and sarcoidosis will cause increased levels. Bone metastasis with resorption from breast, cervical, and prostate tumors may also cause increase in calcium levels.

SIGNS AND SYMPTOMS

- Anorexia, nausea, fatigue
- Constipation
- Polyuria
- Dehydration
- ECG changes
  - Shortened QT interval
  - Depressed T wave
- Bradycardia
- Heart blocks

DIAGNOSTIC FINDINGS

- Serum calcium level >11 mg/dl
- Serum calcium level >12 mg/dl (may lead to coma)
- Serum calcium level >14 mg/dl (may cause death)

Common clinical findings	Patient teaching
Important nursing implications	Serious/life-threatening implications

NURSING MANAGEMENT OF HYPERCALCEMIA

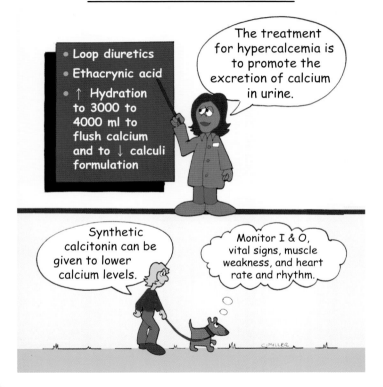

Management of Hypercalcemia

MEDICAL MANAGEMENT

- Administration of IV fluids followed by a loop diuretic (Excretion of calcium is followed by excretion of sodium.)
- Biphosphates (pamidronate) via IV to help reduce bone resorption
- Calcitonin via IV to promote renal excretion of calcium
- Nausea treated with antiemetics
- Stool softeners given for constipation

NURSING MANAGEMENT

- Encourage the client to increase oral intake of fluids to 3 to 4 L/day.
- Institute safety precautions for the client at risk for injury.
  - Be aware of altered gait and weakness.
  - Assess neurologic status every 4 hours—level of consciousness (LOC), orientation.
- Encourage increased mobility.
- Monitor for arrhythmias.
- Monitor IV site for infiltration, erythema, and pain.
- Teach the client to limit intake of foods high in calcium.
- Avoid vitamin preparations that contain vitamin D.

Common clinical findings	Patient teaching
Important nursing implications	Serious/life-threatening implications

HYPOCALCEMIA

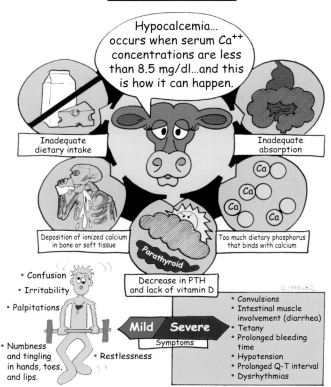

Hypocalcemia... occurs when serum Ca^{++} concentrations are less than 8.5 mg/dl...and this is how it can happen.

Inadequate dietary intake

Inadequate absorption

Deposition of ionized calcium in bone or soft tissue

Too much dietary phosphorus that binds with calcium

Parathyroid

Decrease in PTH and lack of vitamin D

- Confusion
- Irritability
- Palpitations
- Numbness and tingling in hands, toes, and lips.
- Restlessness

Mild Severe
Symptoms

- Convulsions
- Intestinal muscle involvement (diarrhea)
- Tetany
- Prolonged bleeding time
- Hypotension
- Prolonged Q-T interval
- Dysrhythmias

Hypocalcemia

GENERAL

Hypocalcemia can occur as a result of malignancies, vitamin-D deficiency, decreased intake of calcium-containing foods, increased intake of phosphorus (antacids), administration of a large amount of stored blood products, and removal of the parathyroid gland. It may also occur as a result of excessive loss of calcium with the use of diuretics.

SIGNS AND SYMPTOMS

- Tetany—characterized initially by numbness and tingling of the nose, ears, and fingertips (paresthesias) (It may progress to painful muscle spasms and convulsions.)
- Positive Chvostek's sign—twitching of the cheek in response to tapping the facial nerve (Think *C* for Chvostek's = cheek.)
- Positive Trousseau's sign—carpal spasm of the hand when a blood pressure cuff is inflated above the systolic pressure for several minutes
- Hyperreflexia
- Laryngospasm
- Arrhythmias (ventricular fibrillation, torsades de pointes [prolonged QT interval >0.48 seconds])
- ↓Cardiac contractility and ↓BP
- Hypomagnesemia (frequently occurs with hypocalcemia)

DIAGNOSTIC FINDINGS

- Serum calcium level <8.5 mg/dl

Common clinical findings	Patient teaching
Important nursing implications	Serious/life-threatening implications

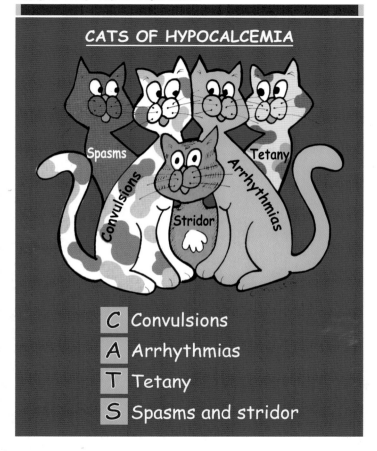

What You Need to Know
Hypocalcemia—CATS

GENERAL
Hypocalcemia can occur as a result of malignancies, vitamin-D deficiency, decreased intake of calcium-containing foods, increased intake of phosphorus (antacids), administration of blood products, and removal of the parathyroid gland.

Using the acronym CATS (Convulsions, Arrhythmias, Tetany, Spasms) helps to establish a triggering device in your memory to bring the symptoms to mind.

SIGNS AND SYMPTOMS
- Convulsions, confusion, paresthesias
- Arrhythmias—ventricular fibrillation, torsades de pointes [prolonged QT interval >0.48 seconds])
- Tetany, hyperreflexia
- Spasms and laryngospasm with stridor
- Positive Chvostek's sign—twitching of the cheek in response to tapping the facial nerve (Think *C* for Chvostek's = cheek.)
- Positive Trousseau's sign—carpal spasm of the hand when a blood pressure cuff is inflated above the systolic pressure for several minutes

Common clinical findings	Patient teaching
Important nursing implications	Serious/life-threatening implications

NURSING MANAGEMENT OF HYPOCALCEMIA

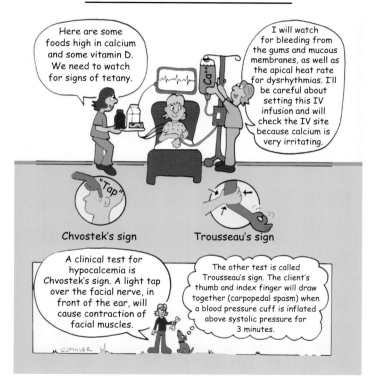

What You Need to Know
Management of Hypocalcemia

MEDICAL MANAGEMENT

For nonacute hypocalcemia:
- Give calcium carbonate PO with vitamin D to help with absorption of calcium in the GI tract.
- The client may need to be given magnesium if serum levels are low.

Emergency management for acute hypocalcemia:
- Administration of calcium gluconate or calcium chloride by slow IV push (0.5-1ml/min)
- Maximum rate for intermittent infusion is 200 mg/min

NURSING MANAGEMENT

- Monitor serum calcium levels every 4 to 6 hours. The goal is to maintain calcium levels between 7 and 8.5 mg/dl (titrate drip accordingly).
- Assess IV site for infiltration:
  - Calcium gluconate and CaCl are damaging to tissue, which can lead to tissue necrosis.
- Monitor cardiac rhythm and ECG changes.
- Assess for ↓ BP.
- Evaluate for presence of paresthesia.
- Check Chvostek's and Trousseau's sign.
- Avoid rapid IV push administration—could lead to rapid drop in BP, arrhthymias, and cardiac arrest.

Common clinical findings	Patient teaching
Important nursing implications	Serious/life-threatening implications

PHOSPHATE

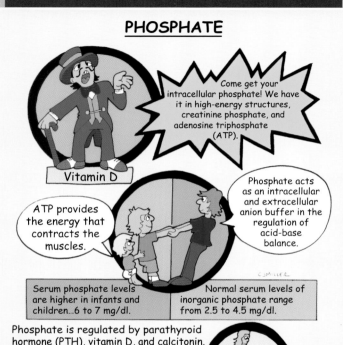

Come get your intracellular phosphate! We have it in high-energy structures, creatinine phosphate, and adenosine triphosphate (ATP).

Vitamin D

ATP provides the energy that contracts the muscles.

Phosphate acts as an intracellular and extracellular anion buffer in the regulation of acid-base balance.

Serum phosphate levels are higher in infants and children...6 to 7 mg/dl.

Normal serum levels of inorganic phosphate range from 2.5 to 4.5 mg/dl.

Phosphate is regulated by parathyroid hormone (PTH), vitamin D, and calcitonin. They work together to determine the daily amount of calcium and phosphate to be absorbed or deposited into the bones and renal absorption or excretion by the kidneys.

↑ phosphate (HPO_4^-) = ↓ calcium (Ca^{++})

What You Need to Know
Phosphate

SIGNIFICANCE OF PHOSPHATE

Phosphate is the most abundant negatively charged anion in the intracellular fluid (ICF) and is essential to the function of muscle, red blood cells, and the nervous system. It is deposited with calcium for bone and tooth structure.

SOURCES OF PHOSPHATE

- Milk, cheese, egg yolk
- Meat, fish, fowl, nuts

CONTROL OF PHOSPHATE

A reciprocal relationship exists between phosphate and calcium (when phosphate is elevated, then calcium is low). Just as calcium needs vitamin D for absorption in the GI tract, so does phosphate. Phosphate is involved as the primary constituent in the mitochondrial energy production of adenosine triphosphate (ATP). (Notice *phosphate* is part of the word.) ATP is used as an energy storage medium for the body.

Maintenance of normal phosphate balance requires adequate renal functioning, because the kidneys are the primary route for phosphate excretion. A small amount of phosphate is lost in the feces.

Parathyroid hormone (PTH) is also important in maintaining normal levels of phosphate by altering the kidney's reabsorption of phosphate and the shift of phosphate from the bones to the plasma.

FUNCTIONS OF PHOSPHATE

- Intermediary in the metabolism of protein, carbohydrates, fats
- Acid-base buffering—binds with hydrogen, which occurs primarily in the urine, making it the primary urinary buffer
- Acidification of the urine
- Muscle contraction
- Transport of fatty acids
- Proper function of red blood cells

| Common clinical findings | Patient teaching |
| Important nursing implications | Serious/life-threatening implications |

HYPERPHOSPHATEMIA

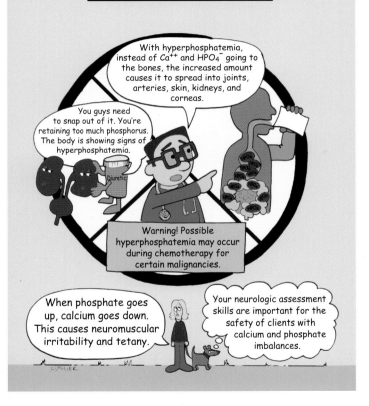

What You Need to Know
Hyperphosphatemia

GENERAL

The major condition that leads to an elevated phosphorus (hyperphosphatemia) in the body is acute or chronic renal failure. Other causes include hypoparathyroidism, increased intake of foods high in phosphorus (milk), excessive use of laxatives or enemas containing phosphate (Fleets enema), large intakes of vitamin D (which increase GI absorption of phosphorus), and chemotherapy for certain malignancies (lymphomas).

SIGNS AND SYMPTOMS

- Reciprocal relationship to calcium—high phosphorus level relates to a low calcium level, leading to hypocalcemia
  - Tetany, twitching of muscles, especially hands and feet
  - Tingling, numbness, cramps
  - Nervousness, irritability, apprehension
  - Anorexia, nausea, vomiting
  - Tachycardia, dysrhythmias, and conduction problems
- Deposition of calcium-phosphorus precipitates in skin, soft tissue, cornea, viscera, blood vessels

DIAGNOSTIC FINDINGS

- Serum phosphorus >4.5 mg/dl (1.5 mmol/L)

Common clinical findings	Patient teaching
Important nursing implications	Serious/life-threatening implications

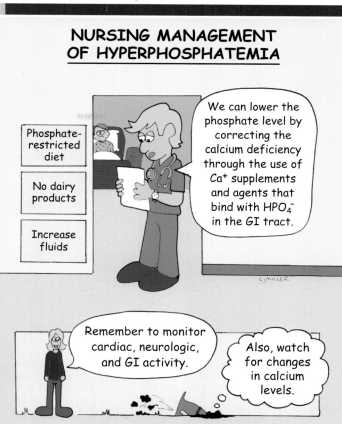

Management of Hyperphosphatemia

MEDICAL MANAGEMENT

- The client should be given vitamin D preparations such as calcitriol (Rocaltrol, in oral preparations), Calcijex (for IV administration), or paricalcitriol (Zemplar) to treat hyperphosphatemia caused by renal failure.
- If hyperphosphatemia is related to volume depletion or respiratory or metabolic acidosis, treat the underlying condition first to correct the phosphorus excess.
- Sevelamer (Renagel) is a binding agent that removes dietary phosphorus from the GI tract.
- Aluminum-based antacids promote elimination of phosphorus from the GI tract (Amphojel).

NURSING MANAGEMENT

- Assess for constipation, which can be caused by taking antacids.
- Assess for signs of hypocalcemia (tetany) because of the reciprocal relationship between phosphorus and calcium.
- Monitor serum phosphate and calcium levels.
- Teach the client to limit foods high in phosphorus—milk, cheese, egg yolk, meat, fish, fowl, and nuts.
- Teach the client that fruits and vegetables are low in phosphorus, especially spinach, rhubarb, bran, and whole grain foods, which may be increased.
- Teach the client to avoid phosphate-containing substances, such as laxatives and enemas.

Common clinical findings	Patient teaching
Important nursing implications	Serious/life-threatening implications

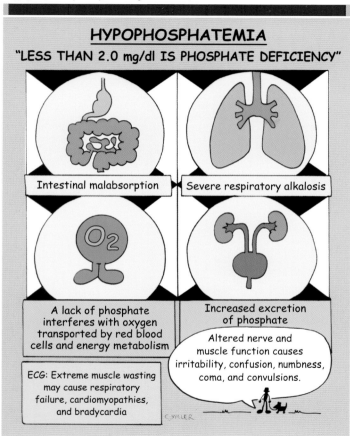

What You Need to Know
Hypophosphatemia

GENERAL
Hypophosphatemia may be caused by increased urinary losses, transient intra-cellular fluid (ICF) shifts, and decreased intestinal absorption. It may also occur with alcoholism, poor dietary intake, vomiting and diarrhea, as well as severe hyperventilation resulting in respiratory alkalosis. Intake of phosphorus-binding antacids (aluminum, magnesium, or calcium antacids) will cause a depletion of phosphorus.

SIGNS AND SYMPTOMS
Acute symptoms result from a sudden decrease in phosphate; chronic symptoms occur when the loss is gradual.
- Neurologic (acute: confusion, seizures, and coma; chronic: memory loss and lethargy)
- Decreased strength (acute: difficulty speaking, weakness of respiratory muscles; chronic: lethargy, weakness, joint stiffness)
- Decreased myocardial contractility with decreased cardiac output and blood pressure

DIAGNOSTIC FINDINGS
- Serum phosphorus <2.5 mg/dl (or 1.7 mEq/L)
- Moderate: 1 to 2.5 mg/dl
- Severe: <1 mg/dl

SOURCES OF PHOSPHORUS
- Meats, especially organ meats
- Fish, poultry
- Milk and milk products
- Whole grains, seeds, and nuts

Common clinical findings   Patient teaching

Important nursing implications   Serious/life-threatening implications

NURSING MANAGEMENT OF HYPOPHOSPHATEMIA
"TWO LEVELS OF CARE"

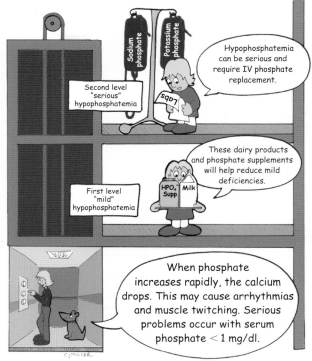

What You Need to Know
Hypophosphatemia

MEDICAL MANAGEMENT

- Mild (1st level)—increase intake of high phosphorus foods
- Moderate (2nd level)—treated with oral phosphate supplements
- Severe (serious)—treated with IV infusion of phosphate

NURSING MANAGEMENT

- Assess and document changes in LOC and orientation.
- Teach the patient that the neurologic changes are temporary.
- Closely monitor the rate of infusion of IV phosphate.
- The patient should be on a cardiac monitor during the infusion of phosphates because of the increased risk of arrhythmias.
- Assess for hypoxemia; patients on ventilators are at higher risk for developing hypophosphatemia.
- Evaluate mobility and the presence of bone pain.

Common clinical findings   Patient teaching

Important nursing implications   Serious/life-threatening implications

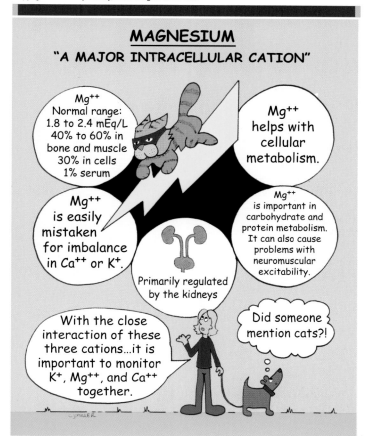

What You Need to Know
Magnesium

SIGNIFICANCE OF MAGNESIUM

Magnesium plays an important role in intracellular reactions, bone metabolism, and action potentials. It activates enzymes for carbohydrate and protein metabolism. It also triggers the sodium-potassium pump and affects the levels of potassium in the cell. It is important in the normal function of the central nervous system (CNS) and in myocardial function.

SOURCES OF MAGNESIUM

- Vegetables (best source)
  - Broccoli, spinach, squash, avocados, potatoes
- Whole grains, nuts, seeds
- Commonly found in tap water, because it is a mineral
- Fruits
- Tuna, pork, chicken

CONTROL OF MAGNESIUM

Although it is not quite understood which organs control levels of magnesium in the body, the kidneys help control high magnesium levels by excreting it through the feces and conserving it by storing it in bone when levels are low. A direct relationship exists between magnesium, potassium, and calcium. This is important because only 1% of magnesium is found in the extracellular fluid (ECF). Serum laboratory values may reveal a normal magnesium level even if a low magnesium level exists.

FUNCTIONS OF MAGNESIUM

- Aids in the synthesis of RNA and DNA
- Cofactor in clotting cascade
- Helps activate B-complex vitamins
- Acts directly on myoneural junction, affecting muscular irritability and contractions
- Maintains strong and healthy bones
- Acts as the transporter for sodium and potassium across cellular membranes
- Cardiovascular regulation by producing vasodilation

Common clinical findings	Patient teaching
Important nursing implications	Serious/life-threatening implications

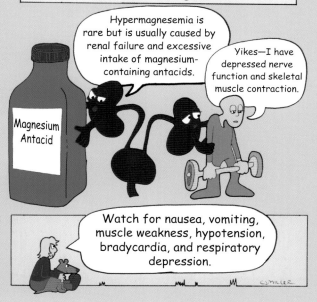

Hypermagnesemia

GENERAL

Occurs with magnesium levels >2.5 mEq/L. This condition is most often seen in clients with renal failure. Decreased muscle activity is seen as a result of a blockage of acetylcholine at the myoneural junction—respiratory muscles may be affected, as well as cardiac conduction.

Hypermagnesemia may also be seen in clients with diabetes mellitus, diabetic ketoacidosis (DKA), or acute lymphocytic and myelocytic leukemia. Patients with leukemia are at increased risk for developing this condition as a result of the nephrotoxic drugs, which directly cause damage to the kidneys leading to renal insufficiency.

Clients who ingest large amounts of magnesium-containing antacids such as Tums, Maalox, Mylanta, or laxatives such as Epsom salt, Milk of Magnesia (MOM), and citrate of magnesia are also at increased risk for developing hypermagnesemia.

SIGNS AND SYMPTOMS

- Muscular weakness
- Diaphoresis
- Hypotension
- Bradypnea
- Decreased deep tendon reflexes
- Flushing
- Decreased level of consciousness (LOC)

DIAGNOSTIC FINDINGS

- Check BUN and creatinine routinely.
- Serum magnesium level is >2.5 mEq/L.
  - When obtaining a blood sample, it is imperative that the sample not be shaken because this may cause hemolysis of red blood cells, which may give a false positive of an elevated magnesium level.
- Serum magnesium level >9 mEq/L is a medical emergency.
  - The client will exhibit absent deep tendon reflexes, decreased LOC, bradycardia, and severe hypotension, which may result in coma and cardiac arrest.

Common clinical findings	Patient teaching
Important nursing implications	Serious/life-threatening implications

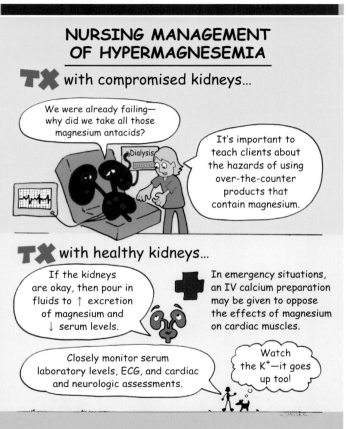

--- **What You Need to Know** ---
Management of Hypermagnesemia

MEDICAL MANAGEMENT

- Administer IV solution containing calcium salts (calcium gluconate) for severe hypermagnesemia.
- Administer diuretics for patients with normal renal function.
- Discontinue use of medications containing magnesium.
- Clients with renal failure may be placed on dialysis.

NURSING MANAGEMENT

- Assess neurologic status for mental status and reflexes.
- Report if the client has absent deep tendon reflexes (especially the patellar reflex) or decreasing LOC.
- Closely monitor intake and output.
- Check skin for flushing and diaphoresis.
- Monitor vital signs; watch for bradycardia and hypotension.
- Provide a list of foods and drugs containing magnesium that should be avoided.
- Client will need continuous cardiac monitoring.
- Report a prolonged QT interval, a wide QRS complex, or the presence of an atrioventricular (AV) block.
- Carefully monitor serum magnesium levels in obstetric clients receiving magnesium sulfate for treatment of pregnancy-induced hypertension (PIH) and preterm labor.
- Evaluate the newborn's magnesium levels if the mother was receiving magnesium sulfate immediately before delivery.

Common clinical findings	Patient teaching
Important nursing implications	Serious/life-threatening implications

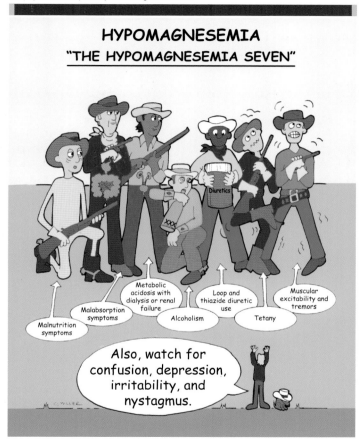

What You Need to Know
Hypomagnesemia

GENERAL

Normal serum laboratory values for magnesium are 1.5 to 2.5 mEq/L. When magnesium levels fall below 1.5 mEq/L, the condition is known as *hypomagnesemia*. It is imperative to know the clients at risk for developing this condition.

This condition may be present in clients with malabsorption disorders such as inflammatory bowel disease (IBD), bowel resection, and in the bariatric population who undergo gastric bypass surgery. Other causes of hypomagnesemia may be seen in the alcoholic client going through withdrawal, because glucose moves into the cell pushing, magnesium into the extracellular fluid (ECF), where the kidneys excrete it.

Hypothyroidism, hyperaldosteronism, and hypoparathyroidism are other conditions that may contribute to this condition.

Clients receiving diuretics, insulin, amphotericin B, and aminoglycosides (such as gentamicin, tobramycin, and neomycin) or nephrotoxic drugs, as seen with many chemotherapeutic agents, are at increased risk for developing hypomagnesemia.

SIGNS AND SYMPTOMS
- Increased neuromuscular ability (secondary to hypocalcemia)
  - Leg and foot cramping
  - Tremors
  - Twitching (positive Chvostek's sign)
- ECG changes: prolonged QT interval, widened QRS complex
- Cardiac arrhythmias (atrial fibrillation and frequent premature ventricular contractions)
- Difficulty swallowing
- Paralytic ileus

DIAGNOSTIC FINDINGS
- Magnesium serum laboratory value is <1.5 mEq/L.
- Calcium levels may be decreased because of decreased action of parathyroid hormone (PTH).
- Potassium levels may be decreased because of failure of the sodium-potassium pump.
- Symptoms may not be seen in the client until magnesium levels are <1 mEq/L.

Common clinical findings	Patient teaching
Important nursing implications	Serious/life-threatening implications

NURSING MANAGEMENT OF HYPOMAGNESEMIA

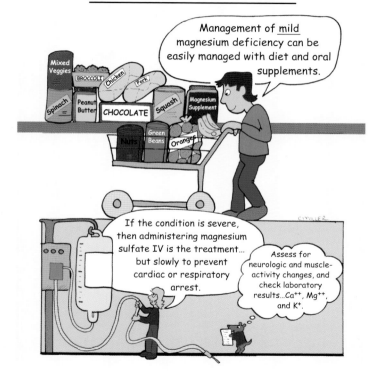

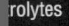

What You Need to Know
Hypomagnesemia

MEDICAL MANAGEMENT

- Replace magnesium either orally or parenterally.
- For oral replacement, the client may be given magnesium oxide tablets, or antacids containing magnesium such as Mylanta or Tums.
- Potassium and calcium levels may need to be corrected.
- For IV replacement therapy, administer magnesium sulfate.
- Infuse magnesium sulfate at a slow rate (<150 mg/minute).
- Never give magnesium as an IV bolus; it may cause sudden cardiac arrest.

NURSING MANAGEMENT

- Obtain a history of the current medications the client is taking. Certain medications may need to be discontinued if they are contributing to the low magnesium levels.
- If the client is on digoxin, check for digitalis toxicity. Hypokalemia potentiates digitalis toxicity.
- If the client is on IV magnesium, check for decreased patellar reflexes, respiratory difficulty, and decreasing blood pressure. Stop the infusion if these occur.
- Assess for presence of dysphagia.
- Assess serum laboratory values for the presence of hypokalemia and hypocalcemia.
- Provide a list of magnesium-rich foods to the client.
- Advise the client that over-the-counter drugs such as diuretics and corticosteroid creams should not be used because they may decrease magnesium levels.

Common clinical findings   Patient teaching

Important nursing implications   Serious/life-threatening implications

---

HYPERCHLOREMIA

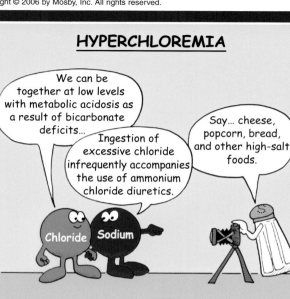

What You Need to Know
Hyperchloremia

GENERAL

One of the primary actions of chloride is to maintain neutrality in relation to sodium and bicarbonate. Hyperchloremia is rare but may occur with a bicarbonate deficiency and dehydration. When a low serum pH exists, the kidneys try to compensate by excreting anions. A loss of anions may result in bicarbonate deficiency and hyperchloremia. Increases and decreases in chloride are proportional to changes in the sodium.

SIGNS AND SYMPTOMS

- No specific symptoms are associated with chloride excess.

DIAGNOSTIC FINDINGS

- Serum chloride level >110 mEq/L
- May see a serum sodium level >45 mEq/L
- May see a decreased bicarbonate level <18 mEq/L.

Common clinical findings   Patient teaching

Important nursing implications   Serious/life-threatening implications

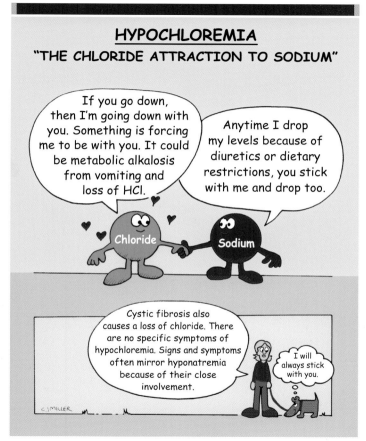

Hypochloremia

GENERAL

Hypochloremia can occur for several reasons. It usually occurs as a result of hyponatremia or increased bicarbonate levels. Vomiting, GI suctioning, and prolonged diarrhea will increase the loss of chloride. Excessive loss of chloride may also occur in cystic fibrosis. Excessive administration of bicarbonates may cause an increase in the bicarbonate levels and a decrease in chloride levels.

SIGNS AND SYMPTOMS

- May be associated with decreased chloride in diet and diuretic use.
- May also accompany hyponatremia, as signs and symptoms often mirror each other.

DIAGNOSTIC FINDINGS

- Serum level <95 mEq/L
- May see sodium serum levels <135 mEq/L
- May see calcium serum levels <8.5 mEq/L

Common clinical findings	Patient teaching
Important nursing implications	Serious/life-threatening implications

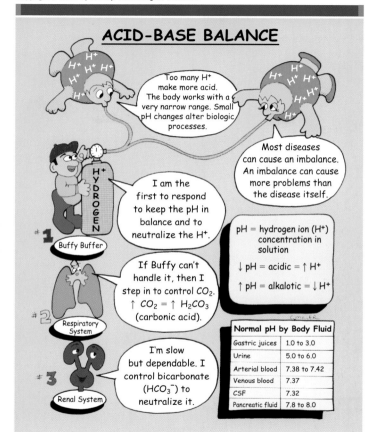

What You Need to Know
Acid-Base Balance

GENERAL

The acid-base balance in the body is controlled by the concentration of hydrogen ions (H^+). The higher the concentration of H^+, the lower the pH and the more acid the solution. The lower the concentration of the H^+, the higher the pH and the more alkaline the solution. Normal body pH is from 7.35 to 7.45. Normal acid-base ratio is 1:20—1 part carbon dioxide (CO_2) to 20 parts bicarbonate (HCO_3). If this balance is altered, then either a state of acidosis or alkalosis exists.

CONTROLLERS OF THE pH

1st response: Bicarbonate, phosphate, protein, and ammonium are all present in body fluids and respond immediately to buffer or combine with excess base or acid produced during normal metabolism. This buffering maintains a normal pH. However, the effect of these buffers is limited.

2nd response: The respiratory center of the brain responds to changes in levels of H^+ by controlling the CO_2 via the respiratory response. $CO_2 + H_2O =$ carbonic acid. If too many H^+ ions exist, then the respiratory rate increases to eliminate excessive CO_2.

3rd response: Renal or metabolic system regulates the H^+ by increasing or decreasing the concentration of bicarbonate and by increased excretion of the H^+.

- Acid-base is evaluated by an arterial blood gas analysis.
- Normal blood gas values are as follows:
  - pH—7.35 to 7.45
  - $PaCO_2$—35 to 45 mm Hg
  - PaO_2—80 to 95 mm Hg (reflects respiratory status, but does not contribute to pH balance)
  - Oxygen saturation—95% to 100%
  - Base excess— +/− 2
  - Serum HCO_3^- —24 mEq/L

Common clinical findings   Patient teaching

Important nursing implications   Serious/life-threatening implications

ACIDOSIS

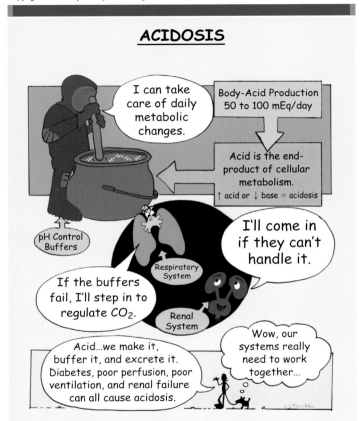

=============== **What You Need to Know** ===============
Acidosis

GENERAL

A state of acidosis exists when the pH is below 7.35. It can be caused by problems in either the respiratory (too much CO_2) or the metabolic system (too little HCO_3).

Respiratory acidosis (retention of CO_2)—neurologic damage (head injury) and/or depression of the respiratory center (anesthesia, narcotics), obstruction of respiratory passages, chronic respiratory problems (These conditions prevent the normal excretion of CO_2 through ventilation.)

Metabolic acidosis—DKA, renal failure, lactic acidosis (shock, cardiac arrest), loss of bicarbonate through diarrhea or intestinal fistulas (In these conditions, an excessive loss of bicarbonate or alkaline fluids is seen.)

Serum potassium (K) tends to go up with acidosis. K moves out of the cells into circulating volume. The kidney tends to retain K as it increases the secretion of H+. When acidosis is corrected, the K will shift back into the cellular compartment.

Compensatory mechanism—Both the kidney and the lungs have a compensatory mechanism to assist the other organs when problems occur. The compensatory mechanism attempts to restore the 1:20 ratio of acid to bicarbonate and return the pH to within normal limits.

If the compensatory mechanism is successful in returning the pH to normal, it does not mean the primary problem causing the imbalance has been resolved.

- If respiratory acidosis is the problem, then the kidneys will compensate by retaining more HCO_3 to balance the acidosis.
- If metabolic acidosis is the problem, then the lungs will increase excretion of CO_2 to assist the elimination of H+ ions and balance the acidosis.

Common clinical findings	Patient teaching
Important nursing implications	Serious/life-threatening implications

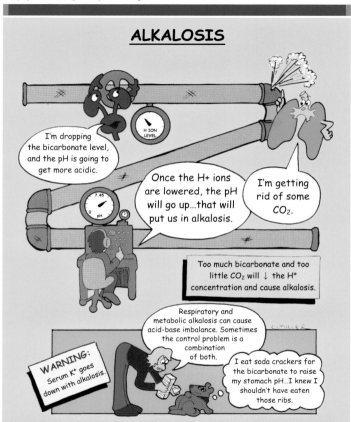

═══════ **What You Need to Know** ═══════
Alkalosis

GENERAL

A state of alkalosis exists when the pH is above 7.45. It can be caused by problems in either the respiratory (too little CO_2) or the metabolic system (too much HCO_3).

Respiratory alkalosis (loss of CO_2) tends to occur when people are nervous and breath too rapidly and diminish their CO_2. It may also be caused by CNS problems affecting the respiratory center, causing hyperventilation.

Metabolic alkalosis—This is an excessive retention of bicarbonate or loss of acid. It may occur if too much bicarbonate has been given during a resuscitation. It may also occur with gastric suctioning or prolonged vomiting and diarrhea.

Potassium (K) tends to go down with alkalosis. K moves into the cells, and increased renal excretion of K occurs as the renal system tries to conserve the H+. If alkalosis is corrected, K will shift out of the cells and back into the circulating volume.

Compensatory mechanism—Both the kidney and the lungs have a compensatory mechanism to assist the other organ when problems occur. The compensatory mechanism attempts to restore the 1:20 ratio of acid to bicarbonate and return the pH to within normal limits (7.35 to 7.45).

If the compensatory mechanism is successful in returning the pH to normal, it does not mean the primary problem causing the imbalance has been resolved.

- If respiratory alkalosis is the problem, then the kidneys will compensate by excreting more HCO_3 to balance the pH.
- If metabolic alkalosis is a problem, the lungs will retain more CO_2 to balance the pH.

Common clinical findings	Patient teaching
Important nursing implications	Serious/life-threatening implications

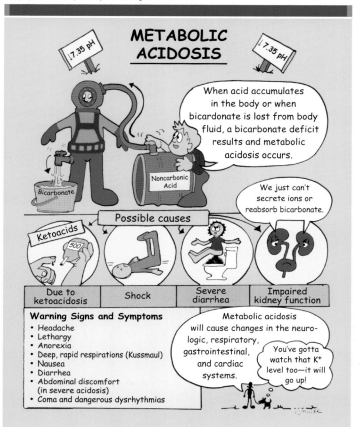

— What You Need to Know —
Metabolic Acidosis

SIGNIFICANCE OF METABOLIC ACIDOSIS

- Occurs as a result of excess acid production in the body or rapid excretion of bicarbonate from the body
- Metabolic system primary problem, respiratory system compensates

COMMON CAUSES OF METABOLIC ACIDOSIS

- Diabetic ketoacidosis
- Lactic acidosis (shock, respiratory or cardiac arrest)
- Renal failure
- Liver failure
- Severe diarrhea
- Vomiting
- Salicylate toxicity
- Starvation
- GI fistulas

SIGNS AND SYMPTOMS

- Kussmaul respirations (deep, rapid respirations)
- Confusion, disorientation progressing to coma
- Headache, lethargy
- Hypotension
- Arrhythmia changes secondary to hyperkalemia associated with diabetic ketoacidosis
- Warm to hot, flushed skin
- Abdominal pain

DIAGNOSTIC FINDINGS

Arterial blood gas results will show the following:

- pH <7.35
- HCO_3 <22
- PCO_2 may be normal (35 to 45 mmHg) or respiratory compensation may occur causing a decrease in the PCO_2 level.
- Urine pH <6

| Common clinical findings | Patient teaching |
| Important nursing implications | Serious/life-threatening implications |

NURSING MANAGEMENT OF METABOLIC ACIDOSIS

↓ pH Metabolic Acidosis ↑H$^+$

Created by
Loss of base (HCO_3^-), excess H$^+$, or inability of kidneys to excrete H$^+$.

- Loss of HCO_3^- (diarrhea)
- Diabetes, alcoholism (ketoacidosis)
- Lactic acidosis (tissue hypoxia)
- ↓ renal function

Nursing Management

Renal function—check BUN, creatinine, and H & H. Watch hydration status for problems with fluid balance.

Support respiratory function—turn, cough, and deep breathe. Check ABGs, and assess Kussmaul's respirations.

Watch electrolytes—check electrolytes. K$^+$ usually goes up in acidosis; Ca^{++} may go down. Assess for cardiac dysrhythmias. Assess blood sugar levels; they may need to be corrected. Antidiarrheal medications or soda bicarbonate may be given to correct acidosis.

Hang in there, I'm coming to help.

=============== **What You Need to Know** ===============
Management of Metabolic Acidosis

MEDICAL MANAGEMENT
- IV bicarbonate may be administered if arterial level is <21 mEq/L or plasma venous bicarbonate level is <20 mEq/L.
- Check arterial blood gases frequently.
- Correct the precipitating cause of acidosis.

NURSING MANAGEMENT
- Identify and treat the cause!
- Determine the history of the precipitating cause—diabetes, alcohol intake, renal disease, excessive GI fluid loss, lactic acidosis.
- Assess serial laboratory results.
  - BUN and creatinine for renal function
  - AST and ALT for liver function
  - Serum electrolytes (Potassium tends to go up; may fluctuate with treatment.)
  - Blood sugar levels
- Monitor arterial blood gases (ABGs).
  - Check pH <7.35.
  - Check HCO_3 <23.
- Check vitals (including temperature and weight).
- If acidosis is a result of diabetic ketoacidosis, administer insulin. Watch out for hypokalemia during administration of insulin, because this moves potassium into the cells.
- Give antiemetics for vomiting.
- Fluid replacement 0.9% or 0.45% NaCl is given for hydration therapy.
- Antidiarrheals if the cause is from excessive diarrhea.
- Assess skin turgor, urine, and weight for hydration status.

| Common clinical findings | Patient teaching |
| Important nursing implications | Serious/life-threatening implications |

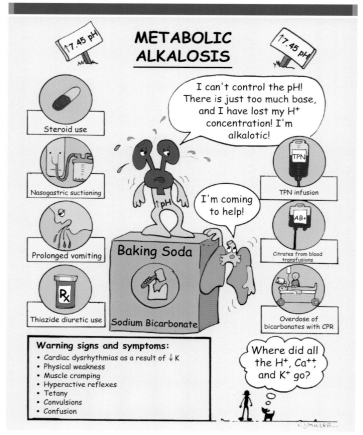

What You Need to Know
Metabolic Alkalosis

SIGNIFICANCE OF METABOLIC ALKALOSIS

Metabolic alkalosis occurs as a result of a loss of acid or a decrease in the level of bicarbonate in the body. The lungs compensate by a decrease in respirations to increase the amount of carbon dioxide (CO_2) in the body by taking fewer and longer breaths. The kidneys also compensate by excreting bicarbonate.

COMMON CAUSES

- Loss of stomach acid through suctioning or vomiting
- Excess alkali intake—antacids, bicarbonate
- GI fistulas
- Adrenal disease (Cushing's syndrome, aldosteronism)
- Diuretic therapy (especially Diamox)

SIGNS AND SYMPTOMS

- Nervousness, dizziness
- Cardiac irritability—($\downarrow$K) ventricular arrhythmias, tachycardia
- Nausea, vomiting
- Paresthesias in the fingers and toes
- Tetany, muscle cramps—late signs
- Hypoventilation
- Assess hydration status—tend to be dehydrated

DIAGNOSTIC FINDINGS

- ph >7.45
- PCO_2 normal or may increase because of compensation
- HCO_3 >28 mEq/L
- Urine pH >6

Common clinical findings	Patient teaching
Important nursing implications	Serious/life-threatening implications

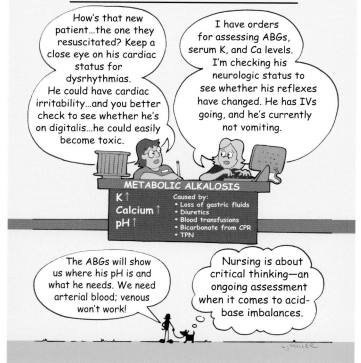

What You Need to Know
Management of Metabolic Alkalosis

MEDICAL MANAGEMENT

- Administration of Diamox increases excretion of bicarbonate.
- Intake of bicarbonate should be stopped.
- Replacement of balanced fluids for patients with GI suctioning, intestinal fistulas, or both is recommended.

NURSING MANAGEMENT

- It is important to determine the underlying cause so that it can be treated.
- Assess for history of precipitating cause—GI suctioning, vomiting.
- Monitor arterial blood gases.
- Monitor potassium values (hypokalemia usually occurs, but levels will increase with treatment of the alkalosis).
- Assess for dysrhythmias—tachycardia and dysrhythmias related to ↓K.
- Monitor respirations (may see bradypnea).
- If the client is taking digoxin, monitor laboratory values. Digoxin toxicity occurs when the serum level is >2.4 ng/ml.
- Give antiemetics to control nausea and vomiting.
- Assess for paresthesias (numbness and tingling) of toes and fingers.

Common clinical findings	Patient teaching
Important nursing implications	Serious/life-threatening implications

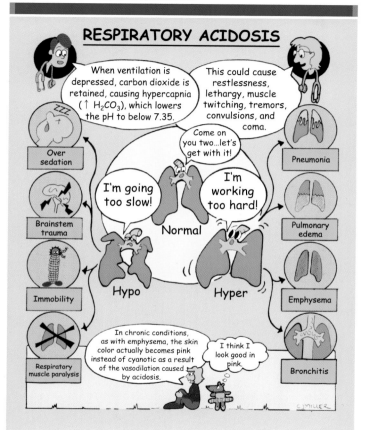

——— What You Need to Know ———
Respiratory Acidosis

SIGNIFICANCE OF RESPIRATORY ACIDOSIS

Respiratory acidosis occurs when there is an excess buildup of carbon dioxide (CO_2) in the blood. It is the most common of the acid-base imbalances.

COMMON CAUSES OF RESPIRATORY ACIDOSIS

Respiratory acidosis occurs secondary to problems that cause hypoventilation:

- CNS depression—head injury, sedatives, anesthesia
- Increased resistance—aspiration, broncho and laryngospasm, prolonged narrowing of airway (asthma, airway edema)
- Loss of lung surface—atelectasis, chronic obstructive pulmonary disease (COPD), pneumonia, pneumothorax, chronic pulmonary diseases
- Neuromuscular diseases—Guillain-Barré, myasthenia gravis
- Mechanical ventilation—increased retention of CO_2

SIGNS AND SYMPTOMS

- Dyspnea, hypoventilation
- Hypoxia
- Restlessness progressing to lethargy
- Drowsiness, confusion, coma
- Tachycardia and tachypnea
- Dysrhythmias associated with hypoxia and hyperkalemia
- Seizures
- Diaphoresis (Skin may appear flushed and feel warm.)
- Hypercapnia ($\uparrow CO_2$) (This will cause cerebral vasodilation and increasing problems with increased intracranial pressure [IICP].)

DIAGNOSTIC FINDINGS

- pH is <7.35.
- PCO_2 is >45.
- HCO_3 may be normal or increased because of compensation.
- Compensation from the renal system is slow.
- Urine pH is <6.

Common clinical findings   Patient teaching

Important nursing implications   Serious/life-threatening implications

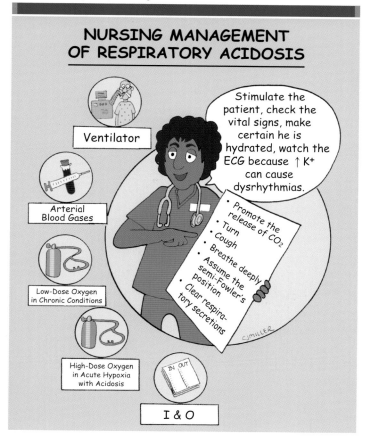

What You Need to Know
Management of Respiratory Acidosis

Even though oxygen does not play a part in acid-base balance, acidosis will occur when the patient does not have an adequate gas exchange. Respiratory suppression, from whatever cause, will precipitate hypoxia (too little oxygen) and hypercapnia (too much carbon dioxide). It is the excess CO_2 that causes the respiratory acidosis.

MEDICAL MANAGEMENT
- Administration of bronchodilators.
- If the client is on a ventilator, the physician may order an increase in the tidal volume to facilitate maximum volume and gas exchange to increase expiration of CO_2.
- Correct the precipitating cause of hypoxia or respiratory problem (if possible).

NURSING MANAGEMENT
- Use semi-Fowler's position to facilitate ventilation.
- Suction as needed (prn) to remove excessive mucus.
- Have artificial airway available.
- Assess patency of airway—respiratory rate, breath sounds.
- Assess for tachycardia secondary to hypoxia.
- Maintain a calm reassuring attitude. (Patients with a decreased respiratory status tend to be very restless and anxious.)
- Teach the patient to use an incentive spirometer.
- Encourage the patient to turn, cough, and deep breathe.
- Monitor patient for bradypnea (respiratory rate <12 breaths/minute).
- Initiate seizure precautions.
- Assess medications. (Sedation may need to be decreased.)
- Encourage ambulation. (Assess patient's response to activity. Stop activity with increasing SOB and tachycardia.)

Common clinical findings   Patient teaching

Important nursing implications   Serious/life-threatening implications

RESPIRATORY ALKALOSIS

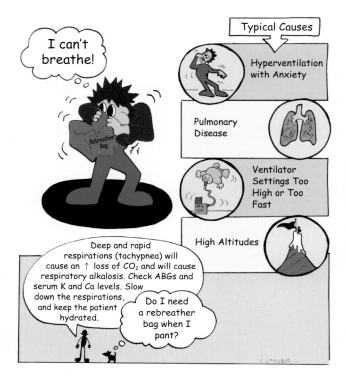

What You Need to Know
Respiratory Alkalosis

GENERAL
This condition is due to low circulating carbon dioxide (CO_2) levels in the blood from hyperventilation secondary to hypoxia, pulmonary emboli, pain, anxiety, pregnancy, or alveolar hyperventilation as seen in clients who are on a ventilator with a high tidal volume and increased respiratory rate.

COMMON CAUSES
- Hyperventilation syndrome (anxiety, hysteria)
- Hyperventilation caused by:
  - Fever
  - Hypoxia
  - Pain
  - Pulmonary disorders
  - CNS problems
  - Assisted ventilation—excessive

SIGNS AND SYMPTOMS
- Hallmark sign is hyperventilation (hyperpnea)
- Client may say he or she feels "light-headed"
- Arrhythmias—tachycardia (potassium may be ↓)
- Anxiety
- Epigastric pain, nausea
- Tetany, seizures, paresthesias in toes and fingers

DIAGNOSTIC FINDINGS
- pH >7.45
- PCO_2 <35
- HCO_3 may be within normal range or <20 if compensating
- pH urine >6

Common clinical findings   Patient teaching

Important nursing implications   Serious/life-threatening implications

NURSING MANAGEMENT OF RESPIRATORY ALKALOSIS

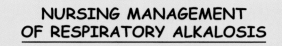

Kidneys help compensate for ↑ pH that is caused by respiratory alkalosis by retaining more H^+ ions.

You can increase the retention of CO_2 by using a rebreather (paper bag) or rebreather mask. Sedatives can also help in a crisis.

As with all acid-base imbalances, it is important to take these nursing actions...

Monitor:
- Respiratory rate and depth
- Tachycardia or ↓ BP
- Serum K levels—cardiac dysrhythmias
- Hydration status—I & O

If the client is on digitalis, then check for toxicity.

=============== **What You Need to Know** ===============
Management of Respiratory Alkalosis

MEDICAL MANAGEMENT

- The client may need to receive an antianxiety medication such as Ativan.
- The physician may order a decrease in the rate and tidal volume if the client is on a ventilator.

NURSING MANAGEMENT

- Identify and correct precipitating cause.
- Monitor arterial blood gases (ABGs)
- Check for presence of ↓ K; monitor for dysrhythmias.
- Try to relax or calm down the patient by providing relaxation techniques such as guided imagery.
- Encourage breathing into a paper sack or rebreathing mask to increase retention of CO_2.
- Reduce environmental noise and stimuli.
- Encourage the client to slow down his or her breathing.
- If the client is having pain, treat it with analgesics.
- If the client is experiencing a fever, treat it.

| Common clinical findings | Patient teaching |
| Important nursing implications | Serious/life-threatening implications |

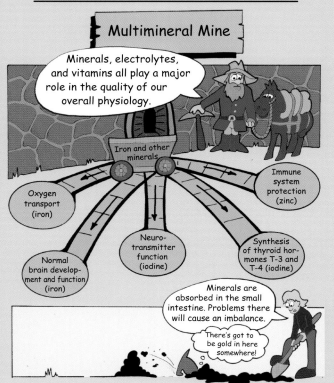

═══ What You Need to Know ═══
Overview of Body Minerals

Iron, iodine, and zinc are minerals found in small amounts in our body tissue. Although the requirements for these trace minerals are small, they are a vital part in maintaining our body functions.

The majority of iron is found in hemoglobin and acts as a transport for oxygen transfer. The presence of vitamin C helps iron to be more readily absorbed. It also helps maintain normal brain development.

Iodine is found in the thyroid gland and works as a temperature regulator; it maintains growth and development of our body working with thyroxine in the thyroid gland, which is a thyroid hormone. It also helps maintain nerve function and metabolism in the body by helping synthesize the thyroid hormones T3 and T4.

Zinc regulates secretion of calcitonin from the thyroid gland and influences bone turnover. It helps stabilize RNA and DNA structure. It also has beneficial properties on our immune system by increasing levels of T lymphocytes to prevent microorganisms and bacteria from causing illness in our body.

Common clinical findings	Patient teaching
Important nursing implications	Serious/life-threatening implications

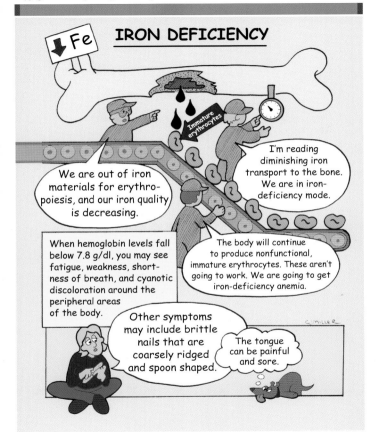

What You Need to Know
Iron Deficiency

GENERAL

Iron deficiency can be caused by a lack of dietary intake of iron. Other factors contributing to iron deficiency are excessive blood loss as seen with GI bleeding, hypovolemia, and malabsorption (or hemolysis). Chronic blood loss is the most common cause of iron deficiency anemia.

- Pediatric implications of iron deficiency—Normal-term infants have adequate iron storage for the first 5 to 6 months; premature infants may need an iron supplement at 2 to 3 months. Toddlers who drink more than 16 to 24 oz of milk are at risk for developing iron deficiency. In addition to not having much iron in it, cow's milk decreases how well the body absorbs iron from other foods. Toddlers who drink a lot of milk tend to feel full and probably are not eating many foods containing iron. Adolescents are at risk because they are growing rapidly and have increased iron requirements. Girls who have started their periods, especially if they have heavy menstrual blood loss, are also at increased risk of iron deficiency.
- Older adult implications of iron deficiency—poor dietary intake and decreased absorption in the small intestine should be considered.
- Pregnancy implications—Diversion of iron to the fetus for erythropoiesis, blood loss at delivery, and lactation can cause iron deficiency.

SIGNS AND SYMPTOMS

- Pallor
- Glossitis (inflammation of the tongue)
- Fatigue, weakness
- Cheilitis (inflammation of the lips)
- Intolerance to cold temperatures
- Headache, paresthesias
- Severe anemia—shortness of breath, dyspnea on exertion, tachycardia, and palpitations, which can progress to cardiac decompensation
- Chronic anemia in children—leads to growth retardation
- "Spoon nails" (nails that develop in a concave shape) or vertical ridges

DIAGNOSTIC FINDINGS

- Hemoglobin levels <7 to 8 g/dl and hematocrit <21% to 24%
- Platelet count >450,000

Common clinical findings	Patient teaching
Important nursing implications	Serious/life-threatening implications

IRON EXCESS—HEMOCHROMATOSIS

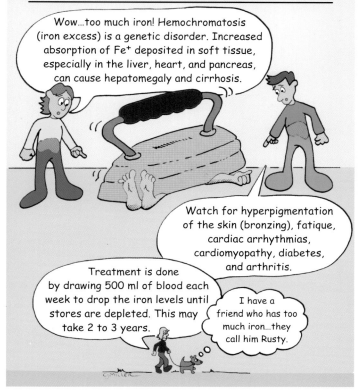

Wow...too much iron! Hemochromatosis (iron excess) is a genetic disorder. Increased absorption of Fe⁺ deposited in soft tissue, especially in the liver, heart, and pancreas, can cause hepatomegaly and cirrhosis.

Watch for hyperpigmentation of the skin (bronzing), fatigue, cardiac arrhythmias, cardiomyopathy, diabetes, and arthritis.

Treatment is done by drawing 500 ml of blood each week to drop the iron levels until stores are depleted. This may take 2 to 3 years.

I have a friend who has too much iron...they call him Rusty.

What You Need to Know
Iron Excess—Hemochromatosis

GENERAL
This condition is not as common as iron deficiency and is seen more frequently in men than women. It has two forms: (1) genetic and (2) acquired. In acquired hemochromatosis the most common cause is due to excessive blood transfusions or can be secondary to thalassemia. The genetic disorder is an autosomal recessive disorder.

SIGNS AND SYMPTOMS
- Hepatomegaly and cirrhosis
- Diabetes
- Cardiac and liver failure
- Cardiomyopathy
- Bronzing of the skin
- Arthritis
- Testicular atrophy in men

DIAGNOSTIC FINDINGS
- Elevated serum iron
- Liver biopsy is the definitive test for diagnosing the condition

MEDICAL MANAGEMENT
- Removal of iron from the body
- Usually achieved by weekly removal of 500 ml of blood for 2 to 3 years until patient's iron stores are depleted

NURSING MANAGEMENT
- Encourage client to limit intake of foods that are high in iron.
- Monitor vital signs during removal of blood.
- Care associated with diabetes and cardiac failure will also be part of the treatment plan.
- Stress the importance of early diagnosis and treatment.

Common clinical findings	Patient teaching
Important nursing implications	Serious/life-threatening implications

IODINE DEFICIENCY

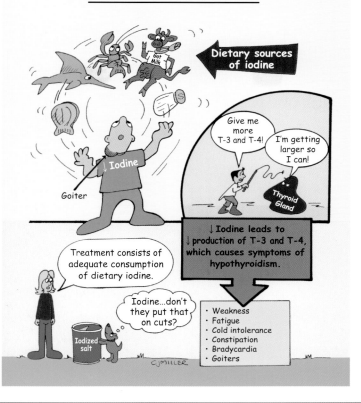

What You Need to Know
Iodine Deficiency

GENERAL
The condition is characterized by a lack of iodine in the body. When thyroid hormones have used up all of the iodine in the body for synthesis of T3 and T4, the pituitary gland recognizes that no iodine exists in the body, so it releases hormones to the thyroid gland to produce more thyroid hormones. Thyroid hormones regulate body temperature, control metabolic rate, and support nerve and muscle function. Inevitably this causes the thyroid gland to enlarge (unilateral or bilateral), which is known as *goiter*. The most devastating complications occur when iodine is deficient during fetal and neonatal growth.

SIGNS AND SYMPTOMS
- Symptoms associated with hypothyroidism—intolerance to cold, dry skin, weakness, lethargy, bradycardia, constipation
- Hyponatremia
- Hoarseness—because of pressure of goiter on the larynx

DIAGNOSTIC FINDINGS
- Decreased T4 and elevated TSH

MEDICAL MANAGEMENT
- Replacement of iodine is achieved most easily by requesting that the client use iodized salt (70 mcg/g) in cooking and at the table.
- Initiate thyroid replacement therapy, such as Synthroid for hypothyroidism symptoms.
- The client may require a thyroidectomy (removal of the thyroid gland) if multinodular goiters are present.

NURSING MANAGEMENT
- Educate the patient on the importance of consuming at least 50 micrograms of iodine daily.
- Provide a list of foods (shellfish, iodized salt, milk, and saltwater fish) that are high sources of iodine, and instruct the client to incorporate these foods in his or her diet.
- Monitor thyroid function studies levels if client is in the hospital.

Common clinical findings	Patient teaching
Important nursing implications	Serious/life-threatening implications

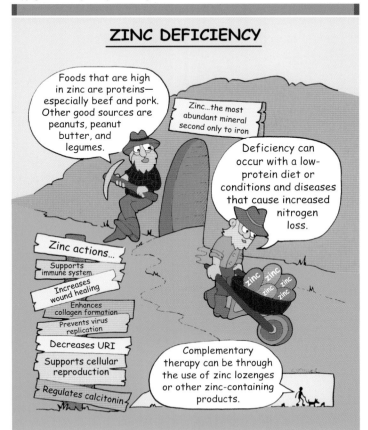

===== **What You Need to Know** =====
Zinc Deficiency

SIGNIFICANCE OF ZINC

Zinc deficiency may result in suppression of the immune system and cause an increase in infections. It is important to the normal functioning of the immune system and assists to prevent replication of viruses. Deficiency may be caused by low dietary intake or by injuries/conditions that cause tissue destruction and increased nitrogen excretion, which also increases excretion of zinc. Intake may be increased in severe inflammatory GI conditions or extensive wounds such as burns.

CLINICAL USE

Zinc, vitamins A and C, and iron are given to facilitate optimal wound healing. The dose of these elements may be higher than the recommended daily allowance.

It may be used to prevent upper respiratory infections, to facilitate wound healing, and for prevention of skin disorders.

Supplements are available in oral tablets, lozenges, or gel application to mucous membranes (not recommended to take over 15 mg/day).

Coffee, bran, and calcium may decrease absorption.

Common clinical findings	Patient teaching
Important nursing implications	Serious/life-threatening implications

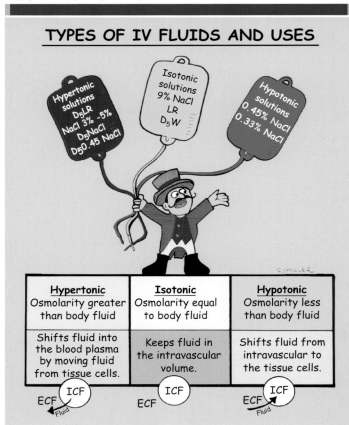

TYPES OF IV FLUIDS AND USES

Hypertonic solutions
D_5LR
NaCl 3% –5%
D_5NaCl
$D_5$0.45 NaCl

Isotonic solutions
9% NaCl
LR
D_5W

Hypotonic solutions
0.45% NaCl
0.33% NaCl

Hypertonic Osmolarity greater than body fluid	**Isotonic** Osmolarity equal to body fluid	**Hypotonic** Osmolarity less than body fluid
Shifts fluid into the blood plasma by moving fluid from tissue cells.	Keeps fluid in the intravascular volume.	Shifts fluid from intravascular to the tissue cells.
ECF (ICF) Fluid	ECF (ICF)	ECF (ICF) Fluid

What You Need to Know
Types of Intravenous Fluids and Uses

ISOTONIC SOLUTIONS

Isotonic solutions have the same osmolarity as normal body fluids (between 250 and 375 mOsm/L). Because they have the same osmolarity as normal body fluids, isotonic solutions help by expanding the extracellular fluid (ECF) space.

Examples: 0.9% NS; Lactated Ringer's (LR) solution; 5% Dextrose in water (D_5W); 5% Dextrose in 0.3% NaCl and LR

Common Uses: Dehydration; maintenance fluid to keep the veins open with long-term IV administration; intravascular compartment expansion

What to Watch for
- Fluid volume overload
- Low hemoglobin and hematocrit levels because of dilution by overexpansion intravascular compartment
- Dextrose rapidly metabolized, leaving free water to be distributed (This will increase the intracellular fluid [ICF] and may cause cerebral edema.)

HYPOTONIC SOLUTIONS

Because of an osmolarity that is less than normal body fluids, the body fluids will shift out of blood vessels into cells and interstitial spaces. Hypotonic solutions help hydrate the cells and can decrease the amount of fluid in the circulatory system.

Examples: 0.45% NS; 0.33% NS

Common Uses: Lower serum sodium levels; expand and hydrate cells

What to Watch For
- Monitor sodium levels. Patients with low blood pressure should not receive hypotonic solutions because this will drive their blood pressure down even further.

HYPERTONIC SOLUTIONS

Because of an osmolarity that is greater than body fluid, this solution draws fluid out of cells into circulating volume. Hypertonic solutions help to restore circulating volume. An increased risk of intravascular fluid volume overload exists.

Common Uses: Hypovolemia and hyponatremia

What to Watch for: Wet breath sounds; increase in blood pressure; fluctuation of serum sodium levels

Common clinical findings	Patient teaching
Important nursing implications	Serious/life-threatening implications

SELECTING ADMINISTRATION SETS

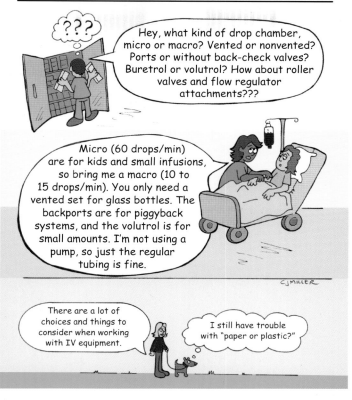

Hey, what kind of drop chamber, micro or macro? Vented or nonvented? Ports or without back-check valves? Buretrol or volutrol? How about roller valves and flow regulator attachments???

Micro (60 drops/min) are for kids and small infusions, so bring me a macro (10 to 15 drops/min). You only need a vented set for glass bottles. The backports are for piggyback systems, and the volutrol is for small amounts. I'm not using a pump, so just the regular tubing is fine.

There are a lot of choices and things to consider when working with IV equipment.

I still have trouble with "paper or plastic?"

=================== **What You Need to Know** ===================
Selecting Administration Sets

TYPE OF CONTAINER

- Glass—Some specialty fluids come in glass containers that are vacuum sealed. These will require vented tubing.
- Plastic—Most standard fluids come in flexible plastic containers. These will require either regular or pedi drip tubing but do not require a vent.

ADMINISTRATION SETS

Drop Size

- Micro (pedi) drip chambers deliver 60 drops/ml.
  - Uses: pediatrics, elderly adults, clients requiring limitations on IV infusion rate
- Macro drop drip chambers deliver 10 to 15 drops/ml.
  - Uses: primarily on adults; can be used to infuse fluids rapidly or to infuse a maintenance fluid (e.g., 125 ml/hour).

IV Ports

Continuous flow sets or lines are designed with a port to infuse secondary (piggyback) fluids, medications, or both.

Tubing

All tubing will require "priming" before connecting it to the patient. There should be no free air in the IV tubing.

IV Filters

These filters are required for administration of blood. Check for institution policies related to specific medications requiring filters (not a universal requirement).

Flow Control Devices

Roller Clamps: These clamps regulate the flow of fluid by pressure on the tubing.

Accessory Devices

These regulatory devices surround the tubing and control the drip rate more effectively than the standard roller clamp.

IV pumps

These pumps have the highest degree of accuracy. Examples would be IV infusion of hypertensive or hypotensive medications, total parenteral nutrition (TPN), and administration of fluids for infants and newborns.

Common clinical findings	Patient teaching
Important nursing implications	Serious/life-threatening implications

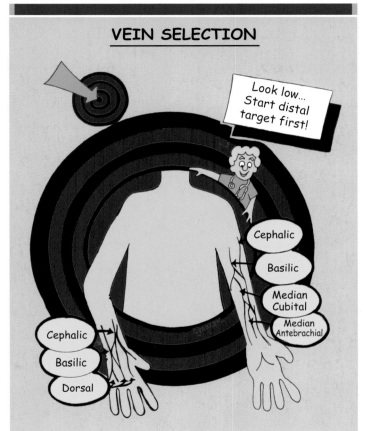

Vein Selection

NURSING IMPLICATIONS

- Verify the order for the rate of IV fluid delivery.
- Check for allergies to iodine solutions or other solutions used to cleanse the skin.
- Verify patient with two forms of identification.
- Teach the client to be careful about using the arm with the IV.

VEIN SELECTION

- Begin with inspection of the distal veins of the hands and arms.
- It is preferable to use a vein on the patient's nondominant side.
- Examine the cephalic vein in the hand and forearm and the median veins of the forearm.
- A vein should be straight and not previously used for IV insertion.
- Palpate the vein; it should be soft, full, and unobstructed.
- Avoid areas where valves exist in the veins (seen as small nodules in the vein). It is sometimes difficult to thread a catheter through a vein valve.
- Select a vein that is appropriate for the type of solution and catheter required—larger veins for blood or IVs that will stay in place for several days and for infusion of irritating fluids. For example, potassium and antibiotics are very irritating to tissue.
- Veins in the hands are suitable for "butterfly" needles and short-term therapy.
- Avoid the following:
  - Areas of flexion
  - Areas of previous infiltration or phlebitis
  - Veins on a surgically compromised limb (e.g., patient who has just had a mastectomy)
  - Veins on side of the body that have been neurologically compromised (e.g., cerebrovascular accident [CVA])
  - Veins in an extremity where circulation is compromised

Common clinical findings	Patient teaching
Important nursing implications	Serious/life-threatening implications

VENIPUNCTURE DEVICE SYSTEMS

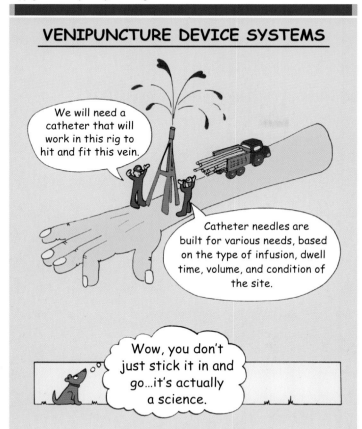

We will need a catheter that will work in this rig to hit and fit this vein.

Catheter needles are built for various needs, based on the type of infusion, dwell time, volume, and condition of the site.

Wow, you don't just stick it in and go...it's actually a science.

What You Need to Know
Venipuncture Device Systems

WINGED CATHETERS (BUTTERFLY NEEDLE)

These catheters consist of a stainless steel needle with soft pliable "wings" on either side to stabilize the needle in the vein.

Use: catheters are used for short-term infusion of fluids or IV push medication.

OVER-THE-NEEDLE CATHETERS

The catheter is a hollow tube that is threaded over the top of a needle or stylet. The needle is used to puncture the vein; blood appears in the flashback chamber when the vein is entered, and the catheter is then threaded over the needle into the vein. The flexible catheter is left in the vein. The Centers for Disease Control (CDC) recommend changing every 96 hours.

Use: catheters are commonly used to infuse IV fluids over several hours to days.

INSIDE-THE-NEEDLE CATHETERS

The catheter is a hollow tube that is inside the needle. The needle is larger than the over-the-needle catheters and is more traumatic on insertion.

Use: catheters may be used for central lines placed in the subclavian vein.

CATHETER GAUGES

The smaller the number, the larger the catheter and needle diameter.

- 24 to 26 gauge may be used on infants, elderly
- 22 gauge—most commonly used for general IV infusion
- 14 to 18 gauge—emergency situations or when large amount of fluid must infuse rapidly

NURSING CONSIDERATIONS FOR SELECTION OF IV DEVICE

1. Amount of fluid and how long it will be infusing
2. Viscosity of fluid (Blood will infuse through a 22-gauge needle, but it will infuse more rapidly through a 20-gauge needle.)
3. Size and condition of the vein (The smallest catheter that will provide the flow rate should be ordered.)

Common clinical findings	Patient teaching
Important nursing implications	Serious/life-threatening implications

IV INFUSION PUMPS

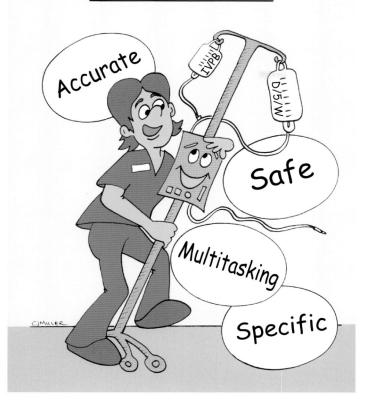

==
What You Need to Know
Intravenous Equipment and Infusion Regulation Devices
(Intravenous Pumps)
==

IV pumps are used in virtually all clinical settings.

MECHANICAL GRAVITY DEVICES

The nurse manually sets the infusion rate on a dial or control device (roller clamp or other type of control device) that is located on the line. These devices are used in outpatient settings, but the nurse must confirm the flow rate by counting the number of drops infused in 1 minute and multiply that by 60 to determine the volume infused in 1 hour.

ELECTRONIC INFUSION DEVICES

These IV devices are commonly used today in the hospital setting. The IV pump calculates the flow rate. There are alarms to recognize an occlusion, air in the line, or a low battery and will sound if one of these issues occurs. Following is a list of commonly used electronic infusion devices:

- Controller—only works by gravity flow
- Positive pressure infusion pumps—can deliver high volumes (used in traumas and intensive care units ([ICUs])
- Volumetric pumps—can deliver small volumes and are used in pediatric, neonatal settings (They require special tubing and can be costly.)
- Peristaltic pumps—used for administration of tube feedings, because this pump periodically squeezes the IV tubing
- Syringe pumps—used to deliver antibiotics and drugs that are to be infused in small-volume amounts (These pumps are limited to deliver a volume that is the size of the syringe.)
- Patient-controlled analgesia (PCA) pumps—can be used as epidural, continuous, or patient- controlled delivery in which the client pushes a button attached to the pump to control administration of medication

Different types of IV pumps can have single or multichannel pumps to deliver several drugs at the same time. Disposable pumps are also used in some ICU settings but are expensive because they must be replaced after each IV administration.

| Common clinical findings | Patient teaching |
| Important nursing implications | Serious/life-threatening implications |

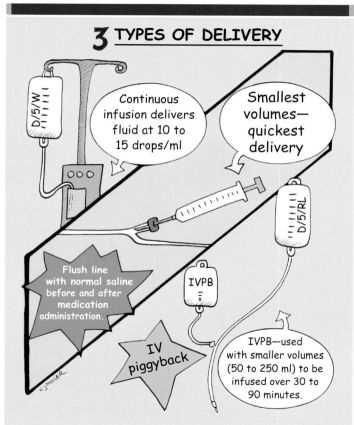

3 TYPES OF DELIVERY

Continuous infusion delivers fluid at 10 to 15 drops/ml

Smallest volumes— quickest delivery

D/5/W

D/5/RL

Flush line with normal saline before and after medication administration.

IVPB

IV piggyback

IVPB—used with smaller volumes (50 to 250 ml) to be infused over 30 to 90 minutes.

CJMILLER

Types of Intravenous Delivery

CONTINUOUS INFUSION: This type of infusion is used primarily for IV fluid maintenance, fluid replacement, or both.

Example: D$_5$1/2 NS @ 100 ml/hr

Nursing Management
1. Monitor the IV insertion site.
2. Watch for *infiltration* (coolness with pain, swelling, and tenderness at site) and *phlebitis* (pain, warmth, and red streaks up the arm from the site).
3. Continuous infusions require a lumen that is large enough to withstand large volumes of fluid. A 20- to 22-gauge peripheral IV catheter, peripherally inserted central catheter (PICC), or central line catheter are preferred. In an emergency or when blood needs to be infused, an 18-gauge may be preferable.
4. Only add fluids to a hanging maintenance bag of fluid if they are to be infused at the same rate as the primary infusion (e.g., potassium and vitamins). If a significant amount of the fluid has already infused, check with the health care provider as to when he or she wants the medication to be started or if the amount of the medication needs to be decreased based on amount of fluid remaining to be infused.

IV BOLUS: This is used to deliver a drug quickly (often in emergency or code situations). It can also be used for a fast response as needed with pain control.

Example: Fentanyl, 25 mcg IV bolus every 30 to 60 min, as needed for pain.

Nursing Management
1. Flush the line before and after delivery of the drug.
2. Check compatibility of the drug with what is already infusing in the line.
3. Instruct the client to report any of these symptoms: redness, warmth, or numbness at the IV insertion site.

INTERMITTENT INFUSION: IV piggyback (IVPB) is commonly used when administering an antibiotic or electrolyte replacement.

Nursing Management
1. If using an IVPB, a secondary line is required.
2. IV tubing should be changed at least q72h for all IV fluids and drugs.
3. If the medications contain lipids, change q12h to prevent the line from clotting.

Common clinical findings	Patient teaching
Important nursing implications	Serious/life-threatening implications

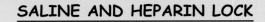

SALINE AND HEPARIN LOCK

Indwelling access ports...

Normal saline

Heparin flush—100 units

...their names reflect the fluid used to keep them open.

Normal saline or heparin keeps the cannula from clotting when fluid is not infusing.

Ships use ports too...

CJMILLER

What You Need to Know
Use of Saline Locks

SALINE LOCKS

Saline locks are used to prevent an IV insertion site from clotting when IV fluids are not infusing.

Nursing Management

1. Check the institution policy and verify the type of line in place.
2. Check patency of the line and lock by flushing it with 1 to 3 ml NS.
3. Patency and blood return can be assessed by gently withdrawing on the syringe.
4. On flushing, check the area distal to catheter end for any discomfort or swelling.
5. Administer medication.
6. Flush the line again with 1 to 5 ml of NS, depending on institutional guidelines.

HEPARIN LOCKS

Heparin is used to prevent an IV insertion site from clotting when it is not being used.

Nursing Management

1. Remember the SASH method:

   Saline—Flush lock with 1 ml of saline.

   Administer medication.

   Saline flush again to clear lock.

   Heparinize with solution of heparin 10 to 100 U/1ml to reseal the lock.

2. Check institution guidelines for heparin lock maintenance. Note the amount and concentration of heparin used to flush and maintain the line. If the line is requiring several milliliters to flush and it is done frequently during the day, the nurse may need to draw back several milliliters of fluid from the line before administering a medication. If not performed, over a 24-hour period, the client can receive a significant amount of heparin.

Examples

- Dialysis catheter
- Central IV catheters
- PICCs
- Butterfly catheters/needles
- Peripheral IV catheter

Common clinical findings	Patient teaching
Important nursing implications	Serious/life-threatening implications

COMPLICATIONS OF PERIPHERAL IV THERAPY

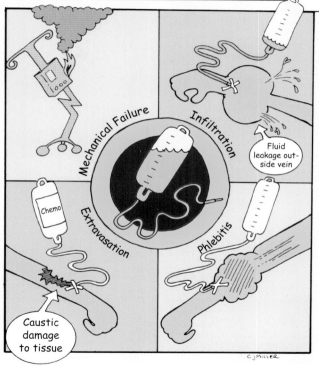

--- **What You Need to Know** ---

Complications of Peripheral Intravenous Therapy

INFILTRATION

Infiltration caused by seepage of IV fluid or medication into surrounding tissue.

Signs and Symptoms
- IV stops infusing or is significantly slower
- Coolness of skin, pain, and tenderness surrounding the site
- Tissue induration and swelling of tissue at end of IV catheter
- Absence of blood return when line is drawn back or fluid container lowered

Nursing Management
1. Assess and document the IV site frequently.
2. Encourage the client to report signs of swelling or pain.
3. Apply warm compresses to infiltrated site, and elevate the site.
4. Follow institution policy regarding whom to notify and restarting of intravenous fluids.

INFILTRATION OR EXTRAVASATION OF CAUSTIC FLUIDS

This is most commonly caused by a medication that causes tissue necrosis in the area of infiltration.

Signs and Symptoms
- Burning, pain at site, inflammation; blisters, sloughing of skin; blanching of skin

Nursing Management
1. Check institution policy regarding removal of an IV catheter. IV antidote may be administered via the present catheter, or the catheter may be removed.
2. Stop the IV; apply cool compresses initially, then warm, moist compresses; elevate the site.

PHLEBITIS

Phlebitis is inflammation of a vein from the cannula, usually because of the length of time the cannula is in, poor-quality peripheral veins. Infusion of irritating antibiotics or potassium will cause inflammation.

Signs and Symptoms
- Redness, pain at site, palpable cord along vein ; warmth around area

Nursing Management
1. Discontinue the IV; apply warm, moist compresses.
2. All peripheral IVs should be changed q72h.

Common clinical findings	Patient teaching
Important nursing implications	Serious/life-threatening implications

CENTRAL VENOUS CATHETERS

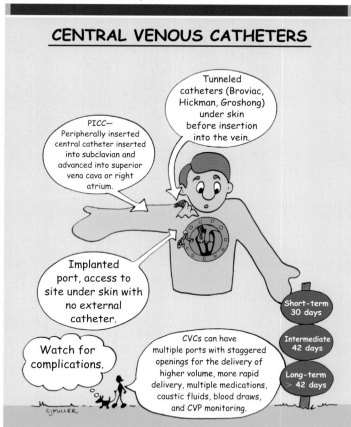

What You Need to Know
Central Venous Catheters

A central venous catheter (CVC) is inserted into the subclavian; it may remain in the subclavian, or it may be progressed into the superior vena cava or right atrium.

These catheters are used for long-term IV access—either continuous or intermittent fluid administration.

- CVC catheters are more stable than peripheral access lines.
- They provide rapid access to high-volume blood flow—administration of blood, hyperalimentation, chemotherapy, and administration of emergency drugs.

TYPES OF CATHETERS

- **Subclavian, midline catheters (MLC)**—single or multilumen lines. The catheter is inserted peripherally in the subclavian area of the neck or threaded from the antecubital fossa. The site depends on the type and length of catheter used and requires heparinization of each lumen if fluid is not infusing continuously.

- **Peripherally inserted central catheter (PICC)**—single or multilumen lines. It is inserted peripherally into the vein at the antecubital fossa and threaded through the vein into the superior vena cava. It requires heparinization if fluids are not infusing continuously.

- **Tunneled catheters** (Hickman, Broviac, Quniton, Groshong) —The catheter is inserted under the skin and tunneled into the superior vena cava. This prevents skin contamination at the site of puncture from contaminating the insertion site of the vena cava. It requires regular heparinizations of the line when fluid is not infusing.

- **Implantable ports** —The catheter is tunneled into place, and a portal or access chamber is sutured under the skin; it may be used for months to years. It is accessed by puncturing the skin over the port with a Huber needle—no external catheter or dressing is required over area when catheter is not in use.

NURSING IMPLICATIONS

1. Consult the institution's policy for dressing changes and irrigating solutions.
2. Check the amount and concentration of heparin used to flush the CVC lines.
3. If an exterior dressing has been used, it is changed under sterile conditions once a day.

Common clinical findings	Patient teaching
Important nursing implications	Serious/life-threatening implications

PEDIATRIC IV THERAPY

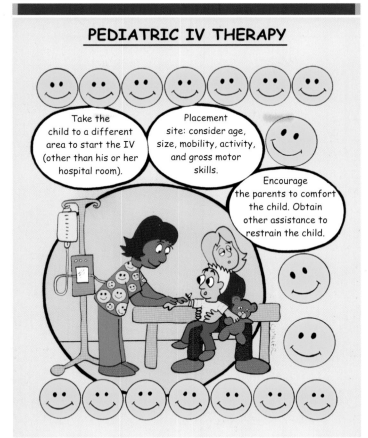

What You Need to Know
Pediatric Intravenous Therapy

Prepare the parents or caregiver before the procedure. Explain to them what you are going to do and the purpose of the IV fluids or catheter.

D_5W should be used with caution in children. It is rapidly metabolized, leaving free water that will increase movement of fluid into the cells, which can result in cerebral edema. NS or LR solution is frequently used for hydration.

BEFORE THE PROCEDURE

- It is preferable to take the child to the treatment room for the procedure.
- Do not ask the parents to help restrain the child during or after the procedure.
- Encourage the parents to comfort the child or infant during and after completion.
- Explain the procedure to the child based on developmental level.

EQUIPMENT

- Volumetric or Buretrol chambers should be used to regulate infusions (if not on an infusion pump).
- Use microdrip tubing (60 drops/ml) to administer a small amount of fluid or medication. Equipment is designed to prevent accidental bolus infusions.

NURSING IMPLICATIONS

1. Monitor fluid balance (I&O, daily weights), vital signs, and LOC.
2. Add supplemental potassium to IV fluids only after renal function has been established.
3. Selection of the site follows same guidelines as for adults.
4. The extremity can be wrapped in a warm pack to increase vasodilation and visibility of the vein.
5. Use a small tourniquet or blood pressure cuff.
6. Do not attempt to start an IV on a child or infant alone; obtain assistance in restraining.
7. Do not tape or wrap all the way around the extremity; this can cause obstruction if swelling occurs.

Common clinical findings	Patient teaching
Important nursing implications	Serious/life-threatening implications